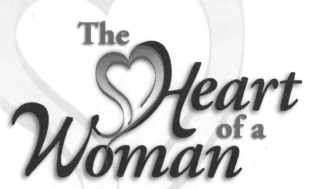

The Heart of a Woman

*A Memoir
of Healing and Reversing
Heart Disease*

Pat Biondi Krantzler, M.A.

Mel Krantzler, Ph.D.

Health Communications, Inc.
Deerfield Beach, Florida

www.hci-online.com

Library of Congress Cataloging-in-Publication Data

The heart of a woman : a memoir of healing and reversing
heart disease / Pat B. Krantzler . . . [et al.].
    p.   cm.
    Includes index.
    ISBN 1-55874-693-5 (trade paper)
    1. Krantzler, Patricia B.—Heart disease in women—
Patients—California—Biography. 3. Coronary heart disease—
Treatment. 4. Mind and body therapies. I. Krantzler,
Patricia B.
RC666.72.K73 A3 1999
362.1'9612'0092—dc21
[B]

                                     99-053982

Publisher: Health Communications, Inc.
           3201 S.W. 15th Street
           Deerfield Beach, FL 33442-8190

Cover design by Larissa Hise
Inside book design by Dawn Grove
Chapter opener illustrations by Genevieve H. M. Wilson, CMI

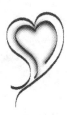

In loving memory of my mother,
Mary Ellen McKillop Biondi,
and my father,
James Edward Biondi,
whose values continue to guide my life.

Contents

Acknowledgments

I wish to acknowledge the warm support I have received from the following members of the TAM and Rehabilitation Staff, who not only helped in my rehabilitation, but also encouraged me to write this book:

Sonja Gumm

Mary Ellen Alesci

Lotte Pons

Alison Jauch

Gary Galloway

Nancy Bloom

And most of all my husband, Mel Krantzler, whose positive reinforcement of my desire to write this memoir made its completion possible.

 # Introduction

In this book, I have chosen to write about my emotional and psychological healing process and renewal of my sense of self in the TAM program, rather than present an overly-detailed technical description of the TAM program, which might have been very boring. It is also the story of the profound changes in my life after I left the TAM program, as well as a backward glance at my life prior to my heart attack.

I have written this memoir of my near-death heart attack and continuing recovery to offer encouragement, hope and enlightenment to the millions of women who are exposed to a similar condition or are in the process of creating their own heart disease without even knowing it.

I was your typical woman—one who had no knowledge that heart disease is the number-one killer of women—and I have paid a devastating price for that lack of knowledge. I invite yo to share in these pages my journey of healing, and reversal of my heart disease in the hope that you can safeguard yourself from such an occurrence, or if you have had a heart attack like mine, you can indeed prevail over it and experience your self-renewal.

1

Prelude

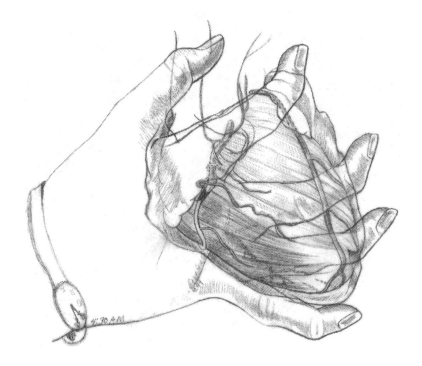

My heart attack began at 4:30 A.M. on Thursday, May 22, 1997.

F. Scott Fitzgerald wrote, "In a real dark night of the soul it is always three o'clock in the morning." For me it will always be 4:30 in the morning.

I woke up startled because it seemed as if I had a very heavy rock in my chest; it had jagged edges and was causing me sharp pains. Sleepily, I placed my right hand on my chest to make the rock disappear, but it didn't. *Must be those tacos and hot sauce I ate for dinner* was my immediate thought.

I glanced at the illuminated clock dial that read 4:30 A.M., still dark outside on a typically mild California morning, a time when all I could hear around me was the deep silence and the heavy sleep of my husband, who was unaware I awoke. I didn't want to disturb him, since it was nothing to worry

3

anyone about—just heartburn that some Maalox
would instantly cure. With that thought in mind, I
walked slowly into my bathroom, which now seemed
like a ten-mile safari although it was only a few yards
from my bed. I swallowed the Maalox and concentrated on walking back to the bedroom feeling shaky
and exhausted, with the rock in my chest—oh, so
heavy!—and sweat on my face and body, and nausea
overwhelming me. I struggled to sit upright on the
side of our bed. The Maalox was not working. *Why
doesn't it work now when it has always worked
before?* I was too weak to lie down again and cover
myself, which I needed to do because an icy chill was
enveloping me. Instead, I slid off the bed and
stretched out on the floor, feeling I was about to faint
and maybe that could cure what I still believed was
heartburn. I did not pass out, and the pain, the nausea, the heavy feeling in my chest and my feeling like
ice continued unabated.

I tried to get up from the floor, but could only
remain kneeling with my hands on the side of the
bed. I had no energy left and it was then that I
semi-shouted, "Mel, Mel, please wake up, I feel so
sick." Mel awoke and looked alarmed. He asked,
"What's the matter, Pat? Why are you on the floor?
What's happening?"

I said it was only a severe case of heartburn and
that the Maalox I took wasn't helping. I did not share
any other detail. Mel wanted to know more, but I kept
repeating, "It's nothing, nothing, it's heartburn and
it's just taking longer to go away, that's all." Mel lifted
me into our bed and covered me. But this had little
effect on my feeling better: I still felt I was at the
North Pole in a nightgown. However, I told Mel,

"Thanks for the help but I'll be my own self again shortly, so why don't you go back to sleep?"

The reason I can write this book is that Mel refused to go back to bed. He once told me jokingly that, when it came to acknowledging I was ill, I was Cleopatra. Why? I asked him. He answered, "Well, you are the Queen of Denial!" A good joke, I thought, but did it really apply to me? It certainly did on that May night.

"Don't call 911!" I screamed when I saw Mel walk out of the room to get to the telephone, for he was concerned, anxious and disturbed over my behavior. He saw the blood drained from my face, the sweat, the grimaces of pain, and questioned whether or not I really had heartburn. But as he told me later, he had no idea I was having a heart attack. After all, I never had such an attack in all my life. I prided myself on being as healthy as a horse. Heart trouble did not run in my family; I had no genetic susceptibility regarding heart disease. So, of course, I kept insisting all I had was heartburn.

I was angry but too weak to resist the call Mel made to 911. (I learned later it was very fortunate Mel called so quickly, because people with a heart attack can die if not taken to the hospital within the first four hours.) I heard him say, "Hurry, please. . . . It's an emergency. . . . Send an ambulance. . . . My wife is very ill. . . . It's her heart."

I was still denying anything was seriously wrong when Mel returned. The last thing in the world I wanted was an ambulance with a screaming siren. Too much commotion for me in my quiet neighborhood. My two Maltese dogs would get upset and start barking like crazy and madly run around the house. I didn't want the neighbors to know I was ill, because it would be very embarrassing.

A terrible fear of hospitals had always been a nightmare of mine, and now the nightmare would become
a reality: I was going to a place that would kill me.
This belief was imprinted in me in the earliest years
of my life. I grew up in a family where money was
scarce. My parents couldn't afford to pay for regular
doctor visits and checkups. My older sister Peggy and
I were supposed to not complain when we were sick,
just stay home and go to bed until we felt better.
Doctor bills had to be avoided. A hospital stay was
out of the question for it would cost a fortune. I knew
that our relatives (who also were poor) only went to a
hospital when they were ready to die from an illness
they experienced without medical care.

My first remembrance of fearing hospitals occurred
when I actually stayed in one, my first and only time.
I was four years old and my parents felt they had no
choice. I came down with scarlet fever, and it was
thought I might have diphtheria, too: a life-and-death
situation for a girl of four. Even today I have vivid
memories of a few flashes from that time. I remember
how fearful I was, asking my parents, "Am I going to
die now that I'm in a hospital?" I remember looking up
at a strange lady near my hospital bed. She was
dressed all in white. Was she the angel of death? I
remember the way she opened and closed my hospital
door without touching the knob and the white rubber
gloves she wore to avoid infecting me. She smiled at
me—a nice smile—when she bent down to pick up my
Mickey Mouse toy that had fallen off my bed and then
brought it back to me the next day all washed and dis-
infected, but the doll didn't seem to look like the one
that had fallen on the floor.

It turned out I only had scarlet fever rather than a
lethal combination with another disease. A narrow

escape. Never again—no more hospitals for me!

(It is no accident I became a psychologist rather than a medical doctor. I have been a specialist in dealing with the psychological problems of my many clients over the past fifteen years. I delight in my work, and nothing makes me feel happier than to help people overcome their problems in interpersonal relationships. But when it comes to physical illnesses, I have always felt helpless. I have always seen myself as a psychologist who heals the psychological, not physical, wounds of others.)

Since the mind is a wild monkey, I once again became that frightened four-year-old girl as I worried about the ambulance arriving with its screaming siren. *Lord, Lord, I hope it doesn't come, maybe they made a mistake about my address. . . .*

However, the ambulance did arrive despite my prayer to the contrary. At first it didn't seem so. I heard a car grinding to a halt; I heard no siren, though, so perhaps it wasn't the ambulance. But it was. (*Why no siren?* was my first thought). Then suddenly I saw three men hastily coming toward me after Mel had pointed the way. They had arrived quickly, just about ten minutes after the 911 call. Mention "heart trouble" and the ambulance service always responds in my city like it is a fire alarm. It was 5:00 A.M. now, and a pleasant-looking man in his late thirties, who said his name was Ted, kept asking me questions: Did I have any pain? When did this start?

Any history of heart problems? He had a kind voice and gentle manner as he took my pulse and blood pressure and felt the sweat on my forehead. I found it hard to talk because I could barely breathe. The pain was so acute, and I told him so. Soon I began to feel better as the pain subsided. (I learned later that Ted and his helpers had given me oxygen, nitroglycerin and some morphine to assuage my pain and the heavy-rock pressure in my chest; he also checked for any changes in my heart rhythm, which would indicate I was having a heart attack. Ted was a paramedic trained in emergency medical procedures, and he could make a basic assessment of a person's illness.)

Since I felt somewhat better, I thought it was the Maalox that was finally working. I then kept repeating, like a mantra, that there really was nothing very wrong with me, just heartburn that was going away. But I remember Ted shaking his head and saying softly, "We can't leave you here, you'll need further checking out at the hospital. It's best for you."

Too weak to protest any further, I suddenly found myself lifted out of our bed and put on a board by the three men present, and then, feeling like a slab of meat, placed in the cavern-like ambulance compartment that was filled with (as I was told later) all kinds of sophisticated equipment: a heart monitor, gel pads for electrodes to be attached to my chest, a blood-pressure cuff attached to my right arm, a nasal prong for oxygen administration, an IV catheter for morphine and nitroglycerin use, and a radio for contact with the hospital. What was being applied to me in the ambulance seemed like a blur at the time. All I remember was that the ride to the hospital was bumpy and that I was viewing everything backward as I lay in the ambulance. Looking through the back-door window I could see dawn emerging and people in their cars beginning their long commutes. As I looked at the cars, I kept thinking enviously: *Here I am going to a hospital while you're going to work. You may hate your job and growl over having to get up so early, but let me tell you I'd rather be in your shoes anytime than in the place where I'm going.*

Seeing everything backwards in the ambulance made things look unfamiliar, and now I was being taken to the most unfamiliar place of all.

The ambulance surprised me by suddenly stopping. *The ride was too short, couldn't it take longer? Must I be taken into the hospital so soon?*

To no avail. The sign said Emergency Entrance, the notice that THE HOSPITAL, like a great beast, was ready to pounce on me. But the morphine was working, diminishing the fear that would have escalated otherwise. Experienced hands quickly liberated me from the jail-like quarters of the ambulance, and soon I was in what looked to me like a larger jail, the hospital's emergency room. I was surrounded by a sudden sea of people in a blur of blue clothing. All I wanted to do was fly away, far away from where I was now, lying on a gurney. Doctors, nurses and technicians seemed to be doing things to me that felt strange and intimidating. All the gadgets they placed on me felt threatening. (I found out later I was on a heart monitor, an EKG to determine my heart elevation, IV catheter, nasal prongs, oxygen mask and morphine.) *Why are they doing this to me? Can't they see I'm getting over my heartburn?* The rock in my chest had disappeared, my breathing felt normal. *So please let me go home! Right now!* (I did not know it was the morphine, nitroglycerin and oxygen that had made me feel better.)

I must have been shouting because the next thing I remember was the up-close face of a doctor, earnestly looking into my eyes as he held my face very gently. In a quiet, firm way he said, "Don't say you have heartburn, dear, you are having a heart attack right now. We see it on the monitor near you. We need all your help to make you better. Are you going to help us?" I said, "Yes," and he said, "Fine."

That moment was the first time I acknowledged the reality of my condition—I never mentioned the word "heartburn" again. Moments later a silent scream of horror reverberated in my head. When I told the doctor, "Yes, I am going to help," I had only half believed it. The little four-year-old girl inside me was crying. *You were lucky when you had scarlet fever,* she was tearfully saying, *but now you are going to die; a hospital is the place where you die, remember that!*

But the little girl was wrong, although I did not know it then. The hospital would in future weeks become the birthplace of my new beginning rather than my end. Yes, I would have died if I had not arrived at the hospital, been diagnosed and operated on within hours of my heart attack. The hospital was not the villain; staying home would have been my killer.

A few minutes later my doctor's voice and the little girl's shock of terror faded away and my eyes felt like lead. The morphine was doing its work and I blanked out. . . .

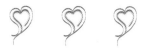

My longest journey into the country of healing and self-renewal began with a single step, which was my recognition that I had survived a very serious heart attack. No longer could I delude myself that it was anything less than that. No longer could I believe, as I had always believed, that women were immune to heart disease, unless they were born with a damaged heart. It was a men-only disease, as so many of my friends who had husbands with damaged hearts also believed.

Letting go of this misconception would enable me to enter the dark forest of the unknown, where my odyssey to survive and discover a new sense of myself would begin. . . .

2

Touch and Go

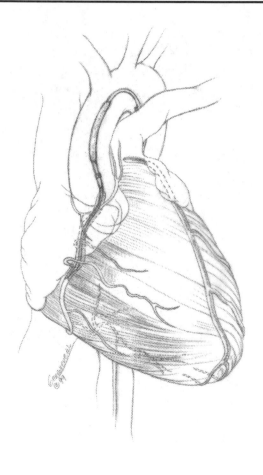

I spent the next eight days in the hospital, but it was more like living in a country called "Nowhere."

I remember that during my hospital stay all I wanted to do was sleep. I remember the nurses, the doctors and the technicians disturbing me, turning me over, taking my temperature and blood pressure. It was a blur of incidents. Why were all those people fussing around and injecting me with God knows what? It seemed that a crowd was always surrounding me, and I felt I was always being disturbed and interfered with. There was no time for me to be by myself. I would hear a voice saying, "It's time to take a blood sample now," which would alarm me. And I remember a sharp voice through the darkness that said, "Don't cross your legs, you'll get a blood clot if you do." Worst of all was my yelling "I can't breathe" and getting angry at the nurse because she wouldn't let me sit up. I was ornamented with plastic tubes and an oxygen mask. It was so annoying, so shameful. I felt so helpless and frustrated, since I had a profound dislike of being waited on or fussed over or told what to do. (Too much of my early life had been spent attending to my mother, who was bedridden

15

from a series of illnesses, including emphysema from working as an accountant in an asbestos-exposed office building, which caused her death.) And I had lost track of time: I had no idea of how long my hospital stay was. Eight days seemed like eight minutes.

Only after I came home from the hospital did I ask my two daughters the details of my stay there. My elder daughter, Karen, a career nurse who has worked in intensive care units as well as in hospices, remained alert about what was happening to me. She was there for me every single day I was hospitalized. Here is what she told me:

> *I was so shaken when I first saw you in that hospital bed. You are my mom, so I didn't want to see you as one of my patients. But I couldn't help noticing how awful you looked. You were really out of it. I don't think during those first days you even remembered seeing me. You were pale, confused and in pain—probably because your heart wasn't pumping the right way—so you weren't getting enough oxygen. The first words I heard from you were, 'I have to get out of here.' But you could hardly speak because your heart was pumping so badly that the fluid would back into your lungs and make you short of breath. Since you weren't getting enough oxygen, you couldn't think clearly.*
>
> *The doctor told me you were in a very unstable condition. He said they didn't know what to do because they would still have to find out how much damage was done to your heart. He told me, 'We'll just have to wait and see.' You had undergone an angioplasty, but they still didn't know how much damage was done to your heart.*

It was touch and go as to whether or not you would even live. You were in critical, unstable condition. Your blood pressure was very low, and because you had a very severe heart attack, your lungs and heart were filling up with fluid from congestive heart failure.

Because the terminology medical practitioners use was a foreign language to me, I would frequently ask Karen, when she was telling me what happened, to explain the meaning of the medical terms she used as a second nature. When she said I had suffered "congestive heart failure," she did not mean my heart failed to beat, but that the way in which my heart pumped was damaged by the heart attack. It meant that my heart wasn't able to get sufficient oxygen and a normal amount of fluid so I could function normally. Karen explained:

That's because you had a lot of blockage in your arteries—those are the blood vessels that carry blood away from the heart to the rest of your body. One artery in particular was all clogged up with plaque, which is fatty deposits that shouldn't be there. When your arteries are blocked, blood flow is reduced, and if there's enough plaque it could kill you by causing your arteries to prevent any blood from flowing. Luckily that didn't happen to you. They gave you an angioplasty very quickly after you entered the intensive care unit— that's known as the ICU—because you were near death. Angioplasty was the procedure you underwent that eliminated the plaque that made it so hard for you to breathe and made your blood pressure so dangerously low.

You were in the intensive care unit for five days, which is far longer than usual—it's the unit where life and death hang in the balance. For most cases, one or two days in ICU is sufficient. But in border-line life-and-death cases it's longer—and you were in that situation. I was so worried because of my background. I probably would have been better off if I hadn't known the things I knew because I was a nurse. It's harder to be a daughter when you know how scary your situation was, Mom. They had clas-sified your condition as critical and unstable.

You were never left alone in the ICU. You received round-the-clock care from three sepa-rate nurses, one for each eight-hour shift. No family member in the first days was allowed to visit you for more than five minutes at a time. You had lots of IV medication. IV means intravenous. The IV is a catheter used to deliver medication intravenously, or directly into the bloodstream through a vein. You had IVs with nitroglycerine, which opens up your arteries so blood could get to your brain, and morphine to relieve your chest pains, and lidocaine, which stabilizes your heart-beat, since your heart was beating in a very irregular way. The monitors in your room showed you had had a heart attack and also how serious it was and if you were improving.

You were right when you remembered that there were lots of people in your room doing all sorts of things to you. You felt they were just annoying you, but really they were a team saving your life. The nurses, the doctors, the medical technicians were all first-rate. They were truly dedicated people. So day by day you were getting better, and on the fifth day they transferred you out of the intensive care unit to a recuperating room. That meant you had graduated—you passed the crisis stage. I felt such a feeling of joy, saying to myself, Thank God, Mom made it!

You spent the next three days in the new room, and it made me so happy that you were improving every day. You could get out of bed, go to the bathroom by yourself, and you could walk in the hall using a walker. Color came back to your cheeks— you were pale as a ghost before, since your blood wasn't circulating properly. You were beginning to look like the mom I always knew. . . .

Vickie, the younger of my two daughters, was also present with Karen at the hospital. She's only fourteen months younger than Karen (raising the two of them was like raising twins!). She's an office manager, and she told me she was glad she knew nothing about the medical details of what was happening to me, like Karen knew. When I questioned her about those eight days I spent in the hospital, she told me:

I was so frightened when I first saw you in the hospital bed. You could hardly breathe and you were white as a sheet

I felt completely at sea. The doctors and nurses paid no attention to me or anyone else in the family. It was as if we shouldn't be there, like we were getting in the way of their work. They should be more sensitive to what the family is feeling. I wasn't there to bother them, I was there to help you. I wasn't just anybody, I was your daughter and you were my mother, and I was there to help in any way I possibly could.

The hospital people told me and Karen that they would tell us about developments with you if we called them up rather than stick around the hospital. We could only see you for five minutes at a time anyway, and, in the beginning, you didn't even know I was there in the room with you!

I was so afraid I would lose you, and then I also got angry at you. I kept thinking, This didn't have to happen, you let things go. You had high blood pressure for a long time, but didn't pay any attention to it, and you continued to smoke even though you knew it was harmful. *I also thought,* How could you do this to me, *as if you were punishing me by being so sick! Then I began to feel very guilty for thinking such wicked thoughts. You were going through a terrible time, so it was wrong of me to think of myself, to be so self-centered. But that was because I loved you so much and couldn't bear the thought you might die right before my eyes, that you might leave me forever. I think I was right, however, about the way the hospital ignored the family. Sure, they gave me a telephone number to get additional information about you, but the line was almost always busy, or the people who were attending to you were not available to come to the phone. It was so frustrating. If the hospital at least would recognize the right of the family to be there and that we needed information so we could help when you came home, it would have been so useful and could have relieved some of my anxiety. But I must admit they did a wonderful job in getting you up and around, and I'm grateful to them for that.*

Vickie was of great help to me during my first week at home after I left the hospital. She took a week's leave of absence and slept overnight at my home to help me, along with my sister Peggy, with all of my chores. She gave me moral support, always reminding me not to give up. I can still see her smiling at me and saying, "You can do it, Mom, you're a strong person." Karen, who lived some distance away, called me each day and give me very helpful advice based on her expertise as a nurse. Ever since my heart attack, they have been there for me when I needed them. This practical and emotional support from my two daughters has speeded up my recovery. To be loved and needed by my children, who volunteer their help without my asking, is a great joy in my life.

On my eighth and last day in the hospital, I was alert enough to be able to think about going home. A quickening sense of excitement came over me as I waited for my husband, Mel, to drive me home. Time, which seemed nonexistent while I was struggling to live, now felt like an endless burden. Each moment of waiting for Mel felt like a year. I was now alert and able to walk by myself. I walked slowly, but I was certain I would be able to resume my old walking pace shortly. At that time my memory was very selective. I told myself I certainly had a tough thing happen to me, but it was only an incident that I would totally recover from once I went home. I would be my old self in no time. The trauma I had experienced (that Karen and Vickie had told me about a month afterward) was hidden from my consciousness at the time I came home from the hospital. I was to learn that my mind, body and emotions were still too vulnerable for me to absorb the enormous threat of being so close to dying. I did not know then that my own sense of self would be dramatically transformed in the next three years. As I write this now, I can smile at that self-deception. "Things are going to be just the same when I go back home," I said to Mel when he came (finally!) to drive me home.

I was to savor this euphoric feeling for the next three days. But then came surprises in the package of my expectations. . . .

READER/CUSTOMER CARE SURVEY

If you are enjoying this book, please help us serve you better and meet your changing needs by taking a few minutes to complete this survey. Please fold it and drop it in the mail.

As a special **"Thank You"** we'll send you news about new books and a valuable **Gift Certificate!**

PLEASE PRINT   C8C

NAME:_____

ADDRESS: _____

_____

TELEPHONE NUMBER: _____

FAX NUMBER: _____

E-MAIL: _____

WEBSITE: _____

(1) Gender: 1)_____Female 2)_____Male

(2) Age:
1)_____12 or under   5)_____30-39
2)_____13-15   6)_____40-49
3)_____16-19   7)_____50-59
4)_____20-29   8)_____60+

(3) Your Children's Age(s):
Check all that apply.
1)_____6 or Under   3)_____11-14
2)_____7-10   4)_____15-18

(7) Marital Status:
1)_____Married
2)_____Single
3)_____Divorced/Wid.

(8) Was this book
1)_____Purchased for yourself?
2)_____Received as a gift?

(9) How many books do you read a month?
1)_____1   3)_____3
2)_____2   4)_____4+

(10) How did you find out about this book?
Please check ONE.
1)_____Personal Recommendation
2)_____Store Display
3)_____TV/Radio Program
4)_____Bestseller List
5)_____Website
6)_____Advertisement/Article or Book Review
7)_____Catalog or mailing
8)_____Other_____

(11) What FIVE subject areas do you enjoy reading about most?
Rank: 1 (favorite) through 5 (least favorite)
A)_____ Self Development
B)_____ New Age/Alternative Healing
C)_____ Storytelling
D)_____Spirituality/Inspiration
E)_____ Family and Relationships
F)_____ Health and Nutrition
G)_____Recovery
H)_____Business/Professional
I) _____ Entertainment
J) _____ Teen Issues
K)_____Pets

(16) Where do you purchase most of your books?
Check the top TWO locations.
A)_____ General Bookstore
B)_____ Religious Bookstore
C)_____ Warehouse/Price Club
D)_____ Discount or Other Retail Store
E)_____ Website
F)_____ Book Club/Mail Order

(18) Did you enjoy the stories in this book?
1)_____Almost All
2)_____Few
3)_____Some

(19) What type of magazine do you SUBSCRIBE to?
Check up to FIVE subscription categories.
A)_____ General Inspiration
B)_____ Religious/Devotional
C)_____ Business/Professional
D)_____ World News/Current Events
E)_____ Entertainment
F)_____ Homemaking, Cooking, Crafts
G)_____ Women's Issues
H)_____ Other (please specify) _____

(24) Please indicate your income level
1)_____Student/Retired-fixed income
2)_____Under $25,000
3)_____$25,000-$50,000
4)_____$50,001-$75,000
5)_____$75,001-$100,000
6)_____Over $100,000

FOLD HERE

((25) Do you attend seminars?

1)_____Yes   2)_____No

(26) If you answered yes, what type?

Check all that apply.

1)_____Business/Financial
2)_____Motivational
3)_____Religious/Spiritual
4)_____Job-related
5)_____Family/Relationship issues

(31) Are you:

1) A Parent?_____
2) A Grandparent?_____

Additional comments you would like to make:

_____
_____
_____
_____

Thank You!!
The Life Issues Publisher
HCI

N-CS

C8C

3

The Wounded Healer

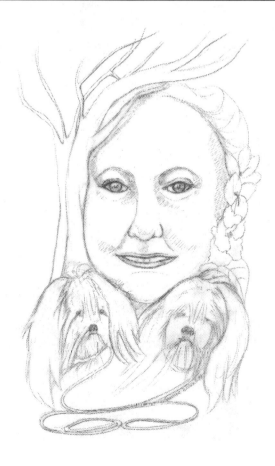

I felt like I was seeing my house for the very first time on the day I came home from the hospital.

I had been living in another reality for eight days that seemed like eternity, bedridden on a ship of death that was nearing its final destination. But now there was a happy ending—just like in the movies. In the nick of time I was rescued by my hero, Dr. Joel Sklar, whose surgical skills saved my life moments before that ship reached port.

Now I returned to the world of the living, but it was not the world I had taken for granted before my heart attack. As I looked around at my house and my garden and trees, the colors were alive as they had never been before. Their intensity almost blinded me: The grass was so vividly green, the garden alive with yellow, red, pink, purple and orange. Even the sky looked different. The clouds were whiter-than-white advancing from a bluer-than-blue background, and the sun shone like newly minted gold.

My two Maltese dogs, Casper and Angie, gave me a joyous barking welcome when I opened the front door of my house. How depressed they were and how lost while I was gone, Mel told me. Now I could enjoy fun times with them again—taking them on long walks, playing games with them, watching them relate to me and Mel and each other. Their liveliness was exhilarating.

My house was saying "Welcome back" when I walked around the rooms like an explorer returning from a threatening foreign country where I couldn't even speak the language. I was again in the familiar environment that I loved.

My initial joy at being home convinced me that what I had experienced in the hospital was just a little "episode," nothing more than that. I told my older sister Peggy (who volunteered to come all the way from Phoenix, Arizona, to help during the first week I came home) that I was now fine, a little weak perhaps, but nothing to worry about. I said to myself, *I'll do everything it takes to remain well: change my diet, exercise daily, lose weight and stop smoking.* I had had a warning lesson, nothing more, so that once I regained my strength I could continue my work and life activities as if nothing happened. But "things" *did* happen three days after I came home that undermined my sense of being in charge of my life as I had always been before.

When I left the hospital I had been given six types of medicine to be used at specific times each day in specific amounts, and warned to always keep nitro-glycerine tablets on hand in case I experienced chest pains again. I was to place a tablet under my tongue. It would relieve the pain and open up blocked blood vessels so my heart could resume normal functioning. The medicine worked well for two days, during which time my sister drove me around Marin County where I lived. We lunched in Sausalito, watching the boats slowly passing by in placid waters, and then spent time visiting the shopping malls. I had to walk a bit slower than usual, but that was to be expected after my operation. Although I was a good driver, Peggy insisted on driving, since she noticed I was still weak. I didn't object. It was such a pleasant and restful visit. And Peggy was a gourmet cook, so I took additional delight in having her prepare meals.

Everything seemed so positive until the third day at home. Upon waking, I felt very nauseated, sick and dizzy. Worse yet, my heart was jumping around like a madman who was erratically banging a drum. I didn't know what was happening, which made it all the more frightening. I panicked and rushed to the phone to call my doctor. He told me to call an ambulance, and forty-five minutes later I was in a replay of that first awful night when I was driven to the emergency room. I was instantly attended to. No, it wasn't a heart attack, but no one knew what it was. Just go home and keep up your regimen as if nothing had happened, the emergency-room staff doctor reassured me. But I hardly felt reassured. In fact, I was scared to death. What if it happened again? Suppose I was driving alone and I felt so nauseated that I lost control of my car? I could crackup in a terrible auto accident, which would be ironic after surviving a near-death heart attack.

I was to experience this horrible panic three more times during my first month home. Five days after the first nausea attack, I had another one, then two more seven days apart. Each time the same symptoms, each time the same call to the doctor, each time the ambulance arriving at my home and whisking me away to the emergency room. It seemed like I was the star and victim of a Halloween play or a *Chicago Hope* rerun. Each time I went through the same routine in the emergency room, and again I was checked and reassured that I had had no heart attack. The emergency-room doctor thought on my third visit that it might have something to do with my medication but made no effort to change my prescription.

On the fourth visit, I broke down and wept hysterically, telling Dr. Sklar it was too much of a strain to undergo this panic, only to come back again and again without finding the source of the problem. But this time he changed my medication. He cut it in half, and that made all the difference in the world in my health and attitude. I began to feel able to stabilize myself and pursue the lifestyle changes that would enable me to become the healthier person I wanted to be. The physical anguish I experienced in that first month was humbling. I had built up a fantasy in my mind that my heart problem was only a minor event that would not interfere with my normal way of life. But now the enormity of the meaning of my heart attack could no longer be denied: It would mean very major, permanent changes in my lifestyle and habits. I would also need to rebuild my self-image, because I had never thought of myself as a victim, a person who waited for things to happen and then responded to them unskillfully. Instead, I always felt I was the person who tried to make positive things happen, a perennial optimist who overcame obstacles instead of wallowing in them. But now my life seemed out of control, making me feel like a victim. As a psychologist, I was familiar with the concept of denial, which is the refusal to accept the reality of a negative traumatic event. Denial can be healthy as a first step toward accepting a shattering event that is initially too painful to face directly. I've seen this happen with many of my counseling patients, such as middle-aged women whose husbands have just died. First they refuse in their minds and emotions to recognize the enormity of this trauma to their lives. They speak of their husband as if he were still alive; they keep his favorite rooms unchanged, as if they were mausoleums; they leave his work desk in the clutter that was always present when he was alive; and his clothes and shoes remain untouched in his wardrobe. Then later on, the new reality that now they must live life as single people emerges into their consciousness. Once they have truly acknowledged the death of their partner—that he is now spirit rather than earth—they begin to rearrange the rooms and to alter the way the house had become a mausoleum. Denial had helped them heal and enabled them to move forward toward renewing their lives in the present, which as their counselor I helped them accomplish.

Now I realized this was exactly what happened to me. It was a continuation of my lack of awareness of my condition during the days I was operated on and cared for in the hospital. I had survived a near-death heart attack, but never knew at that time how near I was to dying.

When I was ready to leave the hospital, Dr. Sklar told me I had undergone a successful angioplasty (which, he explained, was the surgical insertion of a balloon-type plastic-tube catheter into the artery having the most fatty-deposit blockage, called *plaque*). The surgery widened my blocked artery by eliminating the plaque, thus saving my life by allowing me to breathe normally again, since my oxygenated blood could now circulate freely. He also informed me that I had to eliminate smoking (a pack-a-day activity of mine for the past twenty-five years) and to change my lifestyle if I wished to live.

But the mind has a way of protecting itself against very frightening emotions when one is unprepared to deal with them constructively. This is what happened initially when I returned home. At first, I had bliss-fully forgotten I had been an inch away from death and had to change my lifestyle and way of function-ing permanently if I were not to die of another heart attack, which could occur while walking with my dogs in the park, bending down to plant some flow-ers in my garden or vacuuming the floor. In fact, it took that entire first month for me to incorporate that horrifying reality into my consciousness. I had even forgotten the before-going-home meeting with Dr. Sklar, since it meant giving up my smoking habit!

I had always considered myself a realist. "If you're stuck with a lemon, make lemonade out of it" had always been a favorite belief of mine. I had maintained a good track record doing that. Years ago I had endured a traumatic divorce, after which I had to sup-port two young daughters. I was in my mid-thirties, an unskilled housewife with only secretarial skills. Instead of wallowing in self-pity, I went back to college and became a psychologist specializing in inter-personal relationships. I loved my career. I had trans-formed my life and self-image, and in the process of doing so married my second husband, Mel Krantzler, also a psychologist and author. I told my story in a book I wrote with Mel titled *Learning to Love Again.*

I had made lemonade out of the very bitter lemon

of my divorce experience. I always try to communicate this approach to the clients I counsel. If I asked my clients to utilize a crisis in their lives as a stepping stone for their personal growth, rather than as a disaster impossible to overcome, could I ask anything less of myself? The answer was self-evident: Psychologist, heal thyself.

My first step would be moving beyond my denial. That meant gaining as much knowledge about my heart-disease condition as I possibly could. Knowledge is power, and I would need all the knowledge I could accumulate about my heart problem, its prognosis, and the activities and functions I must perform in order to prevent the recurrence of another heart attack. I started by learning about my hospital stay, about which I remembered just that I was surrounded by an impenetrable fog in which I could only recognize vague sounds and movements and physical annoyances. I had no idea where these were coming from. So I sat down with my two daughters, who told me what they saw and heard at the hospital. Even though my condition was touch and go, as they said, I now found it positive to know the details, for knowing how serious it was gave me additional motivation to change my life in ways that would prevent another heart attack.

I remember the day I looked out of my dining-room window at my garden, with its lovely colors enhanced by a vivid noonday sun, and had an epiphany. It was a sudden, intense emotion that reassured me that life is good and that I wanted to live a long time in as positive a fashion as possible. *I'll do everything it takes to make that happen* was the determined shout I heard inside my head.

Along with the powerful feeling that seemed to arise from my soul came the poignant recognition that life is so uncertain. One minute I could be well and the next minute on the edge of death. That realization would challenge me to minimize that kind of risk, to cherish each day as if it were my last, and to free myself from being frightened by the fear of what might happen to me.

These were great resolutions, all of them. But they could easily become the self-deceptions of New Year's resolutions, more honored in the breach than in the practice. T. S. Eliot wrote that between the thought and the act falls the shadow. In my counseling practice, I always had the greatest empathy for my clients who wished to change their self-defeating behaviors but found themselves stuck in the cement of fear of doing something new instead of advancing toward a brighter future. Would I be any different, despite all of my new resolve? Only time and the depth of my motivation to remain alive and well would tell.

I was fortunate to be married to a man who loved me and gave me his entire support in this struggle of mine to renew myself. To paraphrase novelist Ford Madox Ford, Mel has helped me renew my courage and cut asunder my difficulties whenever I've felt ready to throw in the towel in the three years since my heart attack. For despite my natural optimism, at times I became discouraged and fearful, when every step forward seemed to be combined with two steps back. Now, three years after my heart attack, I know from experience that surprises in the disease package can still unnerve you, even though you have positively programmed your life ahead intellectually. I would underestimate the power of my emotions to undermine the good intentions of my intellect.

Mel warned me of this possibility and told me not to be thrown by it. I knew I could rely on his insights and authority, because he himself had experienced a life-threatening disease and could therefore reassure me that I was not going off the deep end in my emotional reactions to my heart attack.

Mel shared with me his own reactions to his life-threatening illness to encourage me that I could triumph over my illness as he had done over his. Some of the things he told me three years ago were things I never knew he felt. Of course, I knew of his prostate cancer, which occurred fifteen years ago, but he had down-played the seesaw of his own emotions. Now, however, he was ready to talk in order to help me successfully manage my own disease. I asked his permission to include what he told me in this chapter.

MEL'S SURVIVAL STORY

Fifteen years ago, in a routine general physical examination, I learned I had prostate cancer. The next day I had a biopsy taken, a very painful surgical procedure, and I remember the doctor saying I had a "nine." I had no idea what "nine" meant, and my ignorance about prostate cancer was total. I naively asked the doctor about that "nine," and the look on his face was grim. He told me the seriousness of prostate cancer was evaluated on a scale of one to ten, ten being highest. My nine was an exceptionally high and virulent number. Later I was given CAT and MRI scans, and the diagnosis was even bleaker: The cancer had metastasized beyond my prostate wall and entered my bloodstream.

The shock I felt on hearing this diagnosis was like having a loaded pistol aimed at my head. Try as I might to keep a bland look on my face, I was emotionally distraught. My whole body felt under attack when I heard this news. I had just had a death sentence leveled at me. "When will the end occur?" I asked the doctor.

He paused, choosing his words carefully. "You do have options," he said. "You could have surgery, excising your prostate, or chemo-therapy, or radiation, or a combination of the two that would not involve surgery. Drugs could also arrest further metastasizing of the cancer." But he refused to give me a time prognosis. Instead, he said a very quick decision was essential. That fact alone was indication enough that I would be lucky to live the year out, and here it was August already.

I heard what I believed was my death sentence, and that night I lay awake for hours. What if I should die in my sleep? Better to stay awake and prevent that from happening. Of course, sheer exhaustion overcame my fear, but when I drifted off to sleep, the dream I had was not reassuring. My dream was literally a running nightmare: a faceless man with a machete was inches away from me as I ran wildly through the streets of San Rafael where I lived. I seemed to have lost my way home.

I woke up relieved; the man with the machete never captured me—almost, but not quite. Sweat had engulfed my entire body; even the sheets on the bed were damp from it. Of course, this dream wasn't difficult to interpret: The man with the machete was the doctor running after me to cut off my manhood.

The doctor as the enemy in my dream didn't surprise me. I had developed, ever since I was nineteen, an intense distrust of medical doctors, particularly surgeons, because my mother died as a result of surgery at that time. She went into the hospital for a minor operation to excise a benign tumor—and died as the result of a blood hemorrhage on the very day she was supposed to return home. She was only forty-one. For years I believed that the hospital people who attended her were incompetent.

So just like Pat, I was uncomfortable in the presence of medical doctors, and chose working as a psychologist with clients who had mental rather than physical problems. Yet now I was burdened with a horrendous medical problem. Was regular contact with hospitals and doctors to become a big part of my way of life?

I, too, lived by the principle of making lemonade out of a lemon. I, however, had always expressed it differently. Being a World War II buff and an admirer of General Stilwell, I try to follow his favorite saying in times of adversity. It was an old Latin saying that he translated as "Don't let the bastards grind you down."

That meant I would fight my disease rather than be victimized by it. I felt life was too valuable to just give up, and my desire for new, challenging experiences was unquenched. Well, the first new challenge was coming to terms with my disease and managing it in such a way that I could live a long time. And even if death would meet me in the next few months, I would live until the moment that occurred.

To accomplish this goal, I had to diminish my obsession with my cancer. *I am not my cancer,* I told myself. *I am, instead, a person who has cancer and can manage it.* In other words, I had the power to make positive things happen in my life, even though I had prostate cancer that would remain with me the rest of my life. When you have a life-threatening disease, it's very easy to believe you *are* the disease, rather than the disease merely being a fact in your life. But there is life ahead for you beyond the disease if you are willing to create it. I had to overcome my distrust of medical doctors and instead learn to substitute a healthy questioning of what they would tell me about my disease. Doctors are not devils or saints; they are men and women, like everyone on this earth, flawed human beings. Their abilities may range from passably competent to exceptional. It was my job to find the very best doctor who could help me live well.

To that end, I embarked on getting second opinions about what I should do: chemotherapy and radiation or surgery? I was fortunate (like Pat) to have some of the very best doctors available and located in Northern California where we lived. Pat was of tremendous help to me at that time, helping me fight my depression and anxiety and attending consultations with the half-dozen doctors I saw, including prostate authorities at Stanford University's hospital, who had international reputations. I was introduced into discovering that doctors don't know everything—and that there is a wide area of "unknowns" that they will acknowledge if you question them closely as I did, because I took nothing for granted. Some of the doctors told me surgery was the best way to enable me to live longer. Others said radiation and chemotherapy. And some even said, "Don't do anything; just wait and see if it gets worse before taking any action." All of these points of view came from the very best experts in the field.

I eventually opted for radiation and chemotherapy under the supervision of a truly fine doctor, Dr. Richard Evans of Marin General Hospital, and a few years later with an equally excellent physician, Dr. Bart Gershbein, in Marin County. Both are also fine human beings who treat me as a person rather than as a disease, and they are the first to admit the wide gaps in knowledge that still exist regarding prostate cancer. Prognosis of the disease and even its development in an individual is still an art more than a science. This does not, however, prevent them from being lifesavers at the time they are most needed. They gave me "hope" as a prognosis, instead of a finite number of months or years to live.

The proof that my prostate cancer did not kill me in three to six months after it was diagnosed (I later learned that usually happened in cases as severe as mine) is that I am writing these recollections *fifteen years* after my original diagnosis. Conventional wisdom would say that I should have been dead long before now, but conventional wisdom is often wrong and must never be

taken as holy writ when we talk about disease—
whether it be cancer, heart disease, or the million
other aches and pains the flesh is heir to.

I have been managing my disease through
radiation initially (five days a week for three
months) and then daily pills and a cancer-arresting
injection and a PSA analysis every three months.
Since the time I was diagnosed, I have written
five other books with Pat's collaboration, and am
now working on my sixth. I have continued with
Pat to counsel people concerning their interpersonal-
relationship problems at our Creative Divorce,
Love & Marriage Counseling Center, and to lecture and teach. I have been acutely aware of the
necessity of maintaininhg an optimistic attitude
to survive a life-threatening disease, such as mine
and Pat's. What happens in one's mind has a
powerful effect on one's immune system and the
direction a disease takes. Fear can eat up the soul
if you let the disease overwhelm your capacity to
think and function. But hope and the determined
desire to prevail over the disease can have enormous positive consequences in mitigating it and
enhancing the quality of daily living.

Pat and I can collaborate on the "wellness"
inherent in our diseases. Our diseases don't
diminish our lives, but represent a challenge to
enhance the quality of our lives in the face of
physical adversity.

When Mel shared with me how he confronted his disease, he also mentioned how I had helped him. I had forgotten that fact. In recalling those anxious times in the first few months after his diagnosis, when I didn't know whether Mel would live or die, I remembered I did reinforce his courage to withstand the assault of his prostate cancer on his mind and body. I had always believed in the mind/body connection that in recent years has received so much positive attention in medical science. Be goal-oriented, keep involved socially with people, think that you will triumph over your disease by managing it, so that even if the disease is present throughout the rest of your life it will not define who you are. Hopelessness is already death-in-life. Realistic hope is life-instead-of-death. Mel told me he never forgot how helpful these words were to him when he had felt depressed.

I began to think of myself as a "wounded healer." I was a person whose career in life as a psychological counselor and writer was to attempt to heal people of their psychological traumas. But now I was the one needing help. I was the counselor who tried to enable people to make positive things happen in their lives, instead of being victimized by events. Now I had a wounded heart and would have to heal my own wounds. The three years following my heart attack would confirm for me many of the psychological developments that Mel experienced in dealing with his prostate cancer, and being able to talk out my hopes and fears with him has been enormously reassuring.

In many ways, my calling myself a wounded healer proved more positive than I initially realized. Native Americans believe that a person who is a healer in

some ways becomes more powerful through awareness of his or her own wounds and vulnerabilities.
Such people can become more compassionate and
insightful about the sufferings of other people and
more understanding of their own survival capacities.
This happened to me during my three years' journey
toward self-renewal through prevailing over the
physical and psychological devastation initiated by
my heart attack. However, I had many miles to go
before this objective could be realized.

I'm reminded of the Chinese saying, "The longest
journey begins with but a single step." My "single
step" was taken when I had my first private visit with
Dr. Sklar shortly after I received the right dosage of
my medication so I could function with an alert mind.

4

I Search for Answers

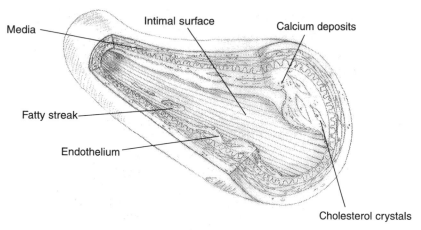

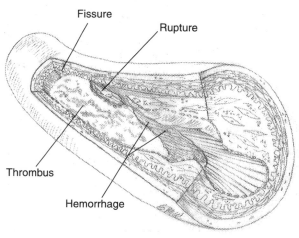

ATHEROMATOUS PLAQUE

I n that first private visit with Dr. Sklar, I discovered him to be a warm-hearted individual as
well as a superb cardiologist. He treated me as a
human being rather than as an illness. Talking with
him made me feel like a partner in a conversation
rather than as a person to be condescended to
because of my ignorance about heart disease.

He told me that my heart problem was indeed serious, but that my angioplasty was a great success and
that he had real hope for my long-term survival. In
fact, I could even reverse my heart disease so that my
quality of life could be vastly improved.

I interrupted him at this point (he had told me to
ask him anything I wanted to know or didn't understand) and asked, "Does 'reversing' my heart disease
mean the disease can be entirely eliminated and that
my heart will be clear of any blockages?"

"That's a very interesting question," he replied. "No,
it doesn't mean that your heart will be clear of any
problems, but it does mean lessening the degree of
blockage that is present in your blood vessels. The
disease you have is called coronary heart disease. It's

the major form of heart disease. It involves blockages in the blood vessels that supply the heart muscle with blood. These blockages that you have are made up of cholesterol and fat and clot and calcium. Reversing these blockages reduces the chance they will cause you to ever have another heart attack. Your heart muscle has been damaged to some degree by partially blocked blood vessels—but the good news is that your heart muscle can be improved and the blockage can be diminished, so you can have a long life ahead of you. You can do this by managing your disease so that the muscle of the heart that isn't damaged can improve through a well-designed program of medication, healthy diet, exercise and stress-reduction changes.

"Think of it this way: You will have to permanently change your lifestyle to make this happen, which means first of all you're never to smoke again—since smoking was the major cause of your heart attack. Any person who smokes is asking for a heart attack, in addition to lung cancer.

"There's a difference between managing a disease—which you will have to do if you want to live—and 'curing' it. Curing a disease means making it go away. But although heart disease can't disappear, it can be managed by you so that your disease is less of a risk. That's reversing your disease so that you'll feel full of life and vigorous in the future."

I had thought that reversing my heart disease meant curing it forever, so I was disappointed in what Dr. Sklar said. But, on the other hand, his explanation was very encouraging in the sense that I could indeed take charge of my illness and not be victimized by it. If I had to "manage" my disease instead of curing it, so be it. But Dr. Sklar said I would have to permanently change my lifestyle. Did that mean taking medication forever? I had always avoided medicine-taking (it reminded me too much of the endless prescriptions my mother took during her long cancer illness). So it was with some trepidation that I asked Dr. Sklar, "Will I have to be medicated forever?"

Dr. Sklar's answer was not exactly reassuring. "No heart patient will probably ever be entirely free of medication," he said. "Even with a change in your lifestyle, it may be that you'll always require medicines to lower your cholesterol or blood pressure, no matter how you manage your life. Blood thinners such as aspirin make a big difference, but can't be eliminated by lifestyle efforts. However, many medications that have side effects can be eliminated—just like they were in your case. You don't seem to have many genetic factors in your family background. That's good, because those can't be managed without medications. Time will tell as to whether or not you'll be able to reduce the amount of medication you're now taking. It's too much to ask to have a disease such as yours that developed over many years simply to disappear once it's gotten a stronghold in your body. So the medicines will always be a part of your life to a greater or lesser degree."

Dr. Sklar was certainly no don't-worry-be-happy dispenser of information. But on second thought, I appreciated his direct answers. He displayed the kind of honesty that respected my intelligence and opened doors to realistic hope for my improvement rather than fantasy hope. In fact, he had praised me for surviving a difficult angioplasty (I could have died if the angioplasty had not effectively opened up my plaque-filled artery). He also said my blood pressure and cholesterol rates were within normal limits as a result of my medication, which augured well for the future. In fact, he sounded genuinely convinced that I could make a reality of that fact. Death could take a long holiday away from me.

The entrance to Dr. Sklar's office listed an organization called Cardiology Associates of Marin & San Francisco Medical Group with his name and those of other specialists itemized below that title. I asked him what Cardiology Associates was. He explained it was an organization of healthcare professionals, of which he was a founding member six years before. All were experts in the field of heart disease in every phase of prevention, surgery, rehabilitation, and reversal of the disease: cardiologists, exercise physiologists, nutritionists, mind/body and stress-management experts, and group facilitators.

"We call our program the TAM Program. TAM means Total Atherosclerosis Management. 'Atherosclerosis' is the hardening of the arteries such as you had. TAM is a holistic approach that treats the whole person, since you're not a disease but an individual," he informed me.

I expressed great interest in what he said. He then gave me a pamphlet that outlined the TAM approach and suggested it could prove very helpful to reversing my heart condition if I wished to join the program.

When I left Dr. Sklar's office, I felt a tingle of hope pass through me—a quickening sense of anticipation that something positive could happen to my health after all. This was the first of my monthly visits with him (now—three years later—I go once every four months), and every time it's been an enlightening and informative experience.

THE TAM PROGRAM©:
A BEACON OF HOPE

When I arrived home that day, one of the first things I did was to read the pamphlet explaining the TAM program. Here is what it said:

The TAM© Approach

TAM stands for Total Atherosclerosis Management. It is an integrated, comprehensive, therapeutic approach to managing atherosclerosis, conducted in a partnership including you, your physician and the TAM Program's staff of professionals.

Recent evidence shows that hardening of the arteries ("atherosclerosis"—the fundamental cause of heart disease) can be prevented, and in many cases, even reversed. These studies confirm the power of the individual to participate in the management of his or her own preventive care, and in fact suggest that the patient's participation is essential to lasting success in cardiac care.

The TAM Program includes all of the key components, including group support, a change in eating habits, exercise, stress management and relaxation techniques. Lifestyle management of atherosclerosis may prevent not only progressive hardening of the arteries, but also heart attacks and the need for angioplasty or bypass surgery.

Risk factors contributing to the process of atherosclerosis can be significantly reduced by changes in your lifestyle. The TAM Program offers individuals with known coronary disease and those individuals with multiple risk factors an opportunity to decrease their risk of progression by adopting new lifestyle skills and habits related to exercise, eating, relaxation and communication.

Stress management, relaxation techniques, and group support will help you learn to deal with such emotions as anger and hostility— which can contribute significantly to high risk behavior.

Your participation in the TAM Program offers you a supportive, integrated environment in which personal growth and positive health changes can occur.

TAM Program© Components

As a participant you will receive:

- Individual and group instruction regarding the less-than-10-percent-fat eating plan
- Computer analysis of your current nutritional status, and follow-up as you progress
- Guidance in shopping, storing, cooking and preparing food for maximum nutritional value
- Stress management and integrated mind/body techniques
- Group support and enhanced communication skills
- Your own cardiovascular fitness plan

How hopeful these words were! What appealed to me most was the emphasis on "the power of the individual" to influence the course of one's heart disease, as well as the specific program components participants would receive. I could hardly wait for Mel to come home so I could tell him about my visit with Dr. Sklar and show him the TAM pamphlet. When he came in, he noticed my excitement and said it was like a day-and-night difference between how I looked that morning and now. I looked so anxious in the morning, but so hopeful now. He read the TAM pamphlet and said, "It sounds great!" I told him I would like to further explore the possibility of becoming a participant in that program, and he gave me his total support.

I called Dr. Sklar the next day and told him I had read the TAM pamphlet and was very much interested in what it had to offer, and when I told him I wanted more detailed information, he invited me to speak with Tana Ripley, who is the program director. The following is a summary of what Tana told me:

The TAM Program was an eight-week course attended by men and women like myself who had experienced heart trouble and had either bypass surgery or an angioplasty and were beginning their recovery. Also included were men and women who were on the verge of having a heart attack and wished to take preventive measures to avoid that happening. The course would start within a week, at which time we would be introduced to the staff, who were all skilled professionals, and would be exposed to the wide variety of activities in the program. . . . It would be a marathon weekend introduction to the course: we would meet on Friday from 6:30 P.M. to 9:30 P.M.

and Saturday and Sunday from 9:00 A.M. to 9:30 P.M.
. . . There would be six men and five women in the
group, who would introduce themselves and explain
why they were in the program. . . . The staff would
also introduce themselves—all were expert professionals in the fields of cardiology, exercise, nutrition
and stress management who would explain their
functions and answer any questions. . . . We would
then have a low-fat dinner prepared by the
Cardiology Associates' chef, Sam, at which time there
would be a summary of what happened that evening.
. . . On Saturday and Sunday we would become
acquainted with the full range of activities an-
nounced the night before. We would view the aerobic
exercise equipment room. We then would have a
group meeting for an hour in which all eleven members would participate and share their personal concerns and expectations about their heart problems.
. . . On both Saturday and Sunday nights we would
again have a low-fat dinner to acquaint us with the
new diet we would need to improve our heart
condition.

After experiencing this marathon, the members of
the group—with professional supervision—would
meet twice a week, on Tuesday and Thursday after-
noon, from 2:00 P.M. to 5:00 P.M. and would utilize all
of the activities they had been exposed to on the
weekend. . . .We would then eat a low-fat dinner from
5:00 P.M. to 6:00 P.M. made in accordance with TAM
principles. . . . The cost of the program then was
twenty-five hundred dollars for the eight weeks and
there would be insurance coverage, since the TAM
Program was the first program of its kind in the State
of California certified by Blue Shield.

I thought the cost was a small price to pay if my life could be saved and my heart disease reversed. Vicki's clear outline of the program excited me, and as she explained it, I could sense her passionate dedication to its goals and her desire to be totally helpful to every person who joined the program. Her work was saving lives that otherwise might be lost. I was to learn that this passionate dedication to saving lives was a conviction every member of the professional staff held. The staff worked as a team and generated an infectious atmosphere of hope to all members of the group.

I told Mel that evening about Vicki's outline of the program, and before I said I really wanted to join, he said, "Go for it!" The next day I signed up. It is the best investment I ever made.

I Learn Some Astounding Facts

The TAM Program would begin in a week, and thinking about it made me want to gain some background information on heart disease beforehand, so I wouldn't be completely ignorant about the subject that was now going to play a paramount role in my life. Where to begin? I have always been a great reader and enjoyed researching subjects that interested me. So my first effort was to visit my favorite local bookstore and screen the wide variety of books in its medical section. The most useful and authoritative book for my purpose was *Mosby's Medical, Nursing and Allied Health Dictionary,* a great, up-to-date book of almost two thousand pages containing clear definitions of thousands of medical terms, which mostly read like a foreign language. I would have to acquaint myself with the heart-disease-related terms if I was to understand what was happening to me. It also had seven useful appendices, including one titled "Leading Health Problems," the subject I was at the moment most concerned about.

When I came home with this book, I first turned to that appendix and was shocked to discover that the leading cause of death in the United States for both men and women was heart disease! It revealed:

> *Cardiovascular diseases (problems affecting the heart and blood vessels) are the leading cause of illness and death for both men and women in the United States. About 44 percent of the deaths in this country are attributable to cardiovascular disease. The majority stems from atherosclerosis.*
>
> *Before menopause women tend to have lower blood pressure and fewer heart attacks than do men of equivalent age. (Female hormones exert a protective effect against heart attacks.) After menopause, the rates among women are higher than those of men and increase with advancing age.*
>
> *The American Heart Association estimates that 69 million Americans have one or more forms of cardiovascular disease.*

I called my daughter Karen and told her I had bought the Mosby book. She said it was one of the best in the field—nurses like herself use it. Since I had always used my computer for research purposes, I asked her what would be the most informative Web site for further information about heart disease. She replied instantly, "The American Heart Association. It's great, all up-to-date material and is written in ways the average person can understand. It's the most helpful I've seen, and has a wonderful listing of linkages."

Karen was right. When I logged on to the American Heart Association Web site, Mel was there beside me. He said he was directly involved in my welfare, and that if he was to be as helpful to me as possible, he would also have to learn the details of heart disease and what I was experiencing. Both of us were astounded at our ignorance once we began to see some of the findings in the AHA newsletters and the reports the AHA sends out on the Internet. Mel and I had thought we were knowledgeable, sophisticated people with advanced university degrees, yet here we were, two beginning schoolkids when it came to knowledge about heart disease. We were to gain the equivalent of Ph.D. degrees in the knowledge of heart disease over the next three years, much of it courtesy of the American Heart Association Web site and its linkages.

By the time I was ready to attend the TAM Program, some of the "truths" I thought I knew about heart disease—particularly about women!—were discovered to be harmful nonsense. Here are some of the "truths" that turned out to be myths:

MYTH: Heart disease is a man's disease.

REALITY: In fact, more women than men die from heart disease. Over a quarter of a million women's lives each year end because of heart disease! One in eight women over the age of forty-five has had a heart attack or stroke!

MYTH: The most serious threat to women's health is breast cancer.

REALITY: Heart disease is women's number-one health threat. Women, however, believe breast cancer is their major threat. (Forty-six percent of women believe breast cancer is their number-one health problem, while only 4 percent believe heart disease is their primary threat!) Heart disease causes double the number of deaths in women than all types of cancers combined!

MYTH: The symptoms of heart disease in women are the same as in men.

REALITY: Women's symptoms are different! Frequent shortness of breath with or without exertion; nausea unrelated to diet; pain or pressure in the chest that comes and goes with or without exertion; trouble breathing; weakness; dizziness; heartburn and nausea—these are usual signs of a heart problem in women, but not in men's heart disease.

MYTH: Scientific studies of heart disease have always included women as well as men.

REALITY: Major studies of heart disease have ignored women! Tests used to detect heart disease are based primarily on studies done on men. Consequently, women are at risk of not having their heart disease detected even though they go to doctors and take the usual (male-oriented) tests.

MYTH: The risk of heart disease in women remains the same whether you are young or old.

REALITY: One in nine women have heart disease between forty-five and sixty-four years of age, while one in three women sixty-five and older have heart disease. After menopause, the risk of having heart disease escalates, since estrogen levels, which protect against heart disease, drop significantly at that time. Since menopause begins earlier now than in previous generations (as early as thirty-eight!), the heart disease risk of the women of the baby-boom generation today is serious indeed; millions of baby boomers are reaching postmenopausal age and their estrogen heart protection is plummeting.

MYTH: Young women who begin to smoke are not at risk of having a heart attack early in life. That can only happen to men.

REALITY: Smoking is the number-one heart attack killer of both men and women. The earlier women smoke, the earlier they may die of heart disease. Smoking is an equal-opportunity killer.

MYTH: Doctors can easily diagnose whether or not a woman has heart disease.

REALITY: Heart disease in women is often overlooked or misdiagnosed by doctors. One-third of all heart attacks in women go unnoticed by doctors because women's symptoms are more subtle than men's. For example, such symptoms of a heart problem in women as having trouble breathing, feeling weak, nausea and heartburn with no chest pain is often misread as having an anxiety attack! A Gallup survey reveals that two-thirds of all primary-care physicians lack understanding of the differences in women's and men's symptoms and diagnoses of heart disease in women.

MYTH: Once you have heart disease or a heart attack you will inevitably die, and die soon, from those afflictions.

REALITY: This is the most dangerous myth of all. It becomes a self-fulfilling prophecy, for if you believe there is no hope at all, you will give up on life, ruin your immune system and die. You will be fulfilling your own prophecy. The good news is that heart disease and heart attacks are not necessarily fatal. In recent times, the remarkable scientific discoveries and curative therapies have validated that heart disease problems, including heart attacks, can be managed as well as reversed in many cases.

As long as such myths exist and are believed, thousands of women each year will be misdiagnosed, or very many women will ignore the real signs that indicate they may have a heart problem. The tragedy is that preventable heart attacks become deaths when this unawareness occurs. I myself had experienced "women's symptoms" that forecast a heart attack without knowing it—heartburn, nausea, weakness—days before my heart attack actually occurred. My survival beat the odds. But there is no reason why we women have to be vulnerable to heart attacks because of a doctor's or our own ignorance. Sometimes we have to educate our doctors.

What I had learned so far about women and heart disease was only the beginning of what now was to be my new lifelong pursuit of knowledge about heart problems. After all, my life was at stake and I was determined to live, but not *just* live. I wanted a high-quality life even if my heart disease could never entirely disappear. Dr. Sklar told me it was definitely possible to manage my disease so that I could lead a relatively active, alert, fulfilling life for many years. Knowledge would be the power engine that motivated me to make this happen.

In this frame of mind, I left my house to attend the TAM Program marathon meeting.

5

I Start the TAM Program©:
The Beginning of
My New Beginning

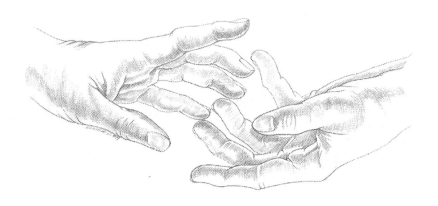

I went to that TAM marathon with a mixture of hopeful anticipation and anxiety. What would it be like? Would people stare at me, point a finger and say, "Shame on you! You've ruined your life and have no one to blame but yourself"?

However, my anxiety turned into pleasant surprise when I opened the meeting-room door and found almost two dozen men and women seated in a circle, looking at me with welcoming eyes. There were six men and five women (including myself), all heart patients who were the new members of the TAM Program. My doctor, Joel Sklar, and his partner Dr. Mark Wexman, codirectors of Cardiology Associates, were also seated in the circle, along with members of their staff: Tana Ripley, R.N., Program Director; Kevin Roberts, Exercise Physiologist; Alan Sadler, Stress Management Consultant; Jan Keating, Dietitian; and Laura Arnold, R.N.

Each of the eleven heart patients in the circle identified himself or herself and almost uniformly said they were there because they had confidence the TAM Program could improve the way their heart was functioning. Four of them mentioned they'd heard of the program from friends who had participated in it and said it helped them enormously—in fact, saved their lives. Some people in the group were referred by their doctors, who encouraged them to participate in the TAM Program because it was the most effective available health-renewal program for heart patients.

I was surprised at the wide variation in ages of the six men and five women in the heart-patient group. Their ages ranged from forty-one to seventy-two. Seated next to me was an airplane pilot who was forty-one years old. Next to him was a seventy-two-year-old priest. There was a forty-five-year-old bank executive, a seventy-one-year-old retired newspaper writer and a fifty-seven-year-old detective. There also was a man of fifty-nine who was not a patient, but the husband of a woman who had just undergone an angioplasty. He joined the group to find out how he could best help his wife by understanding her condition and learning the techniques to help her at home.

All of the five women in the group were of post-menopausal age, in their fifties like I was. (I later learned that the TAM Program had successfully treated women as old as eighty-five in other groups.) All of the women except one had been working outside the home. There was a forensic artist, age fifty-seven, whose husband was attending the meeting; a fifty-four-year-old art appraiser; a college reentry student of fifty-six, who had been working as a full-time secretary and going to school at night to complete her B.A. degree; a fifty-nine-year-old housewife; and myself, age fifty-five, who was a full-time marriage, divorce and family psychological counselor, as well as a writer.

The prominence of so many women in the TAM

Program ended forever the myth I had believed that heart disease was a man's disease, and that I was just an exception to the rule.

As each of us in the group identified ourselves, I noticed we all exhibited a guarded quality, an aura of anxiety mixed with hope. There was a hesitance about sharing too much of one's self, for none of us were then prepared to reveal all of our dark fears and uncertainties—and even panic—about what the future might hold for us. We preferred to demonstrate that we were upbeat, but it was a forced quality, rather than totally authentic. Yes, we wanted to believe that the TAM Program would be effective, but now was a time of watchful waiting, a show-me-it-can-really-happen feeling. As we came to know each other better over the next eight weeks, we would feel much less defensive and would openly reveal more of ourselves and our personal concerns in the group- sharing experience included in each meeting. In fact, some of this tension became alleviated that very first night as a result of the excellent series of orientation talks the Cardiology Associates' staff gave us. After we in the heart-disease recovery group talked a bit about ourselves, each member of the staff outlined the purpose and the goals they had in mind for us. I took extensive notes of each of these professionals' talks and wish to share them with you, for they amount to a short course in heart-disease education and explain the reasons that many different program components were required to successfully accomplish the goal of reversing our heart disease.

Here are the summaries of what each member of the TAM professional staff said:

Dr. Joel Sklar: Why the TAM Program© Is Unique and Successful

Dr. Sklar, with Dr. Wexman, initiated the TAM Program six years ago in Marin County and San Francisco. It was conceived as a team effort in which specialized, scientifically skilled professionals would work together to stop the progression of heart disease and also reverse it. Each patient would have an individual program tailored to his or her heart condition and function in a group rehabilitation setting. Dr. Sklar outlined the TAM approach as follows:

Heart disease technology has vastly improved in the last two decades, and new bypass surgery and angioplasty techniques have resulted in saving hundreds of thousands of lives—four hundred thousand bypass operations and one million angioplasties now occur each year. These men and women are now alive and well, instead of dying as they would have not so long ago. However, all of these new technologies, plus new medicines, were effective only in helping the heart deal better with a blood-flow problem that already happened. It did not answer the most important problem, which was how to stop the progression of the disease or reverse it. That's what the TAM Program is designed to do. We know scientifically that in addition to using the very best medicines—and new discoveries for their improvement are being made all the time— as well as new surgical techniques, permanent lifestyle changes on the patient's part are essential for preventing a second or third heart attack, or a recurrence of plaque and hardening of the arteries. We also emphasize the importance of the mind/body connection. There is now enough scientific evidence to prove that emotions like excessive stress, hostility, anger, despair, anxiety and depression can do as much damage to the heart as smoking, obesity or a fatty diet. Emotions can affect the heart positively as well as negatively. The motivation to permanently change those elements of lifestyle that need changing, the need to see a bright future for oneself, which indeed is possible by making a whole-hearted commitment to the TAM Program—these positive attitudes are great medicine for healing the heart. We are unique in incorporating meditation and Tai Chi, which is a form of meditation through movement, as stress reducers. These techniques are interesting once they are experienced. They're insurance against new plaque formations.

So what we have here at TAM is a combined program that includes the best components, as well as the latest scientific developments, to help heart patients regain their health. The TAM Program is an educational and experiential program designed for getting the mind and attitude adjusted to be able to use the tools learned here. We have an eight-week program, because we know from our past experience it takes that time to incorporate all of the ideas and functions to learn as a part of a new lifestyle. All of us on the staff are involved in the process of teaching how to eat a basically low-fat, vegetarian diet, with some low-fat meat allowed. We don't eliminate fat entirely—it adds taste to food—but we keep it at a minimum. Our dietitian will teach how to monitor new eating habits. Proper exercise comes from a program designed by our exercise physiologist. Our aerobics program is enjoyable, as well as effective in improving the heart. We have a stress-management technique director who educates in the use of stress management to help develop techniques that can help diminish such psychosocial disease-creators as hostility, anger, anxiety and stress. We have a group support and sharing program, because isolation and the inability to share concerns about self, family and work can be very unhealthy. The group can be extremely helpful.

At the end of the eight weeks we hope to see the start of a permanent lifestyle change. The TAM Program is not like taking a test and then forgetting it. It's designed to be a permanent part of life.

After the eight weeks, we have an ongoing graduate program that is voluntary. The purpose of the graduate group is to keep patients focused so that they continue to be motivated and remember all the teachings in the TAM Program. It's a very positive program and reinforces—in a gentle way—patients who have difficulty staying with the program.

We at TAM strongly believe that heart disease is a lifestyle disease. So everyone in the program can have a major impact on healing the heart by changing lifestyle habits. We hope to show how to take personal responsibility to make these habits a permanent part of life. The bonus will be a happier, healthy life, in fact, in many ways a healthier one than the participants have experienced in many years.

Dr. Sklar's talk powerfully reinforced my motivation for joining the TAM Program. He did, after all, save my life with his skillful use of angioplasty to open up my plaque-ridden arteries so I could breathe normally and enable my heart to heal. I was encouraged by his assertion that there was a very real, scientific mind/body connection between toxic emotions like intense stress, anger and depression with heart disease. I had always believed in the mind/body connection when it came to treating my own clients who had stressful psychological problems, so it was supportive for me to know the mind/body connection could also be helpful in healing physical illness.

Dr. Jason Lawrence:
From Skepticism to Belief in the Mind/Body Connection for Healing and Reversing Heart Disease

Dr. Jason Lawrence was a physician with a very interesting story. He had his first heart attack twelve years ago at age forty, but the standard cardiac rehabilitation techniques did not prevent him from having more trouble and a second more severe heart attack. He joined the TAM Program, but with some hesitation, because TAM places great emphasis on stress-reduction techniques as an integral component of the program, aimed at preventing any further progression of heart disease, and perhaps even reversing the disease.

This was a component he initially thought was non-scientific and therefore nonhelpful. So he entered the program with a kind of last-resort-what-do-I-have-to-lose attitude. His testimony to us on his journey from skepticism to belief in the TAM Program, because of its great help in improving his heart condition, generated hope in all the members of the group who heard him that weekend. It was an enlightening educational experience as well as a personal statement. Here is what I recall of his story:

His background had been that of a believer solely in Western scientific thought. So when he was suddenly struck with this heart disease at an early age without having any of the common risk factors, he was skeptical of any explanation other than a so-called medical, scientific one. When stress was named as the culprit causing his disease, his first reaction was that *we all have stress, we all have difficult times in life, so what's the big deal about that? What does the anxiety, frustration and anger I experienced during my years of work and living have anything to do with my heart disease? How do you make a jump from having stress to its causing plaque in my coronary arteries? How could that be an important risk factor?* But he felt he had nothing to lose in working on the stress factor, since everything else seemed to be of little help in diminishing the plaque that could kill him. So he said okay, and worked on reducing stress as aggressively as he worked on the rest of the risk factors that he believed were more scientifically acceptable, like lowering his LDL cholesterol level, the bad kind of cholesterol, and monitoring his diet and exercise. He was interested in finding out whether there was any evidence that the scientist part of him could believe that stress provokes disease, especially coronary heart disease.

It took the TAM Program to personally convince him that the mind/body connection was indeed valid. For, by his active participation in the stress-reduction aspects of the program (meditation through thought and through Tai Chi movement, along with exercise and diet and group reinforcement) he was able to experience what no other program was able to do for him: He was able to prevent his heart disease from progressing, lower his bad LDL cholesterol and stabilize his heart's functioning. He also changed his lifestyle significantly. He was no longer involved in a super-stressful job and overwork, which prevented his nurturing his family life. As he said, his six- and nine-year-old sons now have a real father.

He now affirms the reality of the mind/body connection. His own positive experience of creating a healthier heart for himself through the TAM Program stimulated him to research in depth both the scientific and anecdotal evidence for the validation of this connection. His research amply proved the truth of the mind/body connection. Here is a summary of his major findings, which he shared with the group:

- **On the Nature of Stress:** "When you are talking about stress," he said, "you are talking about perceived stress, stress as your mind perceives it. So what's stressful for me may not be stressful for you. Stress is really a response to something that's an external stimulant. Difficulties at work, arguments at home, money problems, divorce, accidents—these are some of the situations that provoke your perceptions of what stresses you. Therefore, what is perceived is personal.

  "What is also an important component of the deleterious aspects of stress is chronic versus acute episodes of stress. It will turn out that the chronic, unrelenting, persistent factors like anger, hostility, hopelessness, fear, frustration, anxiety and depression are the harmful parts of stress. On the other hand, acute stress, such as seeing a car accident or some disaster on TV news, is an immediate stress that we can't avoid. It's a part of life and can pass quickly. It's when you take a stressful thing with you so that it harbors in your mind—when it persists—that stress can be harmful in a physical way. Studies have shown that stress can prevent the immune system from functioning well. For example, when you are depressed, you are most susceptible to infection because your immune system is functioning poorly." (What he said was that the immune system is in many ways more intelligent than the brain: It has its own way to keep things balanced!)

- **Pain Is a Mind/Body Event:** For example, a long-distance runner seems to tolerate the muscle pain of a marathon with relative ease. That's because of endorphins, which are morphine-like substances that are released in the brain when people run. They alter one's perception of pain and actually provoke a feeling of euphoria, despite the body's being physically exhausted.

- **The Placebo Effect** is another proof of the mind/body connection. Many placebos are simply sugar pills that are given to people in research projects. They are told that the placebo they are taking is a medical pill designed to help treat pain or a specific illness. Many times the illness or pain improves or disappears after taking the placebo because the person *believes* it will work, not because the pill itself has healing abilities.

- **Other Scientific Studies** continue to reinforce the truth of the mind/body connection. Here are some examples:
  (a) Patients with heart disease have more trouble and may have another cardiac problem if they are isolated, angry, depressed or hostile after their first attack. However, if they are in a supportive, caring, group-support system, their mortality rate is better. One clinical study revealed that persons who have heart disease and live in a socially isolated, stressful environment have a *four-times–greater risk of death* in a follow-up three-year period.
  (b) Persons who have undergone angioplasty and have a high hostility level soon have a *two-and-one-half-times–higher* possibility of having clogging or restenosis of the

just-opened artery within six months.

(c) Relaxation techniques have been demonstrated to lower blood pressure in many studies. It's not so much that the relaxation techniques themselves create this effect; instead, it's the *belief* that these techniques can lower blood pressure.

(d) There are several prayer studies which have concluded that intercessary prayer had a beneficial effect on the group of patients prayed for! Here is science and the scientific method applied to the usefulness of prayer in illness.

(e) Anecdotal information validates the mind/body connection: When a loved one dies, the spouse is at greater risk of dying within six months, probably because of hopelessness, depression and despair. There are validated stories of spontaneous remission of diseases like cancer, where the body seems to cure itself or reverse heart disease. No "scientific" reason can as yet account for these occurrences, but there are indications that the mind/body connection generates the remission.

(f) Self-fulfilling prophecies indicate the existence of the mind/body connection. There are stories of voodoo leaders placing curses upon people and saying they will die. No one harms the cursed people, yet they die soon after as the stories go. The voodoo leaders didn't cause the deaths, but the people who were cursed did. The terrible fear effected on the victim, because of the curse, killed the person, not the curse itself. It's possible that the fear translated itself into a physical heart attack.

The conclusions from this mind/body review offered all of us hope. Dr. Lawrence said, "It makes sense to think that if you can worsen a disease process by how you think and feel, then you may also be able to reverse heart disease by changing the way you think and feel."

But he emphasized that this approach in no way diminishes the need for medication, exercise or dietary changes after you experience heart disease. It means, instead, that there is far greater hope for a significant improvement in one's health when all of these factors work in a complementary way to accomplish the same goal—which is a healthier future for everyone in the program.

His speech made me recall an observation from Hippocrates: "It's more important to understand what sort of person has a disease than what kind of a disease a person has. It's the person within that counts the most."

Kevin Roberts, M.S.: The Healing Powers of Exercise

Kevin Roberts, in his words, is an "exercise physiologist." He told us, "I design and implement exercise regimes based on doctors' prescriptions. That takes the form of doing an initial evaluation of what you personally need—what your limitations are—and also to encourage you to enhance your exercise potential.

You will find yourself capable of not only improving your ability to exercise, but also enjoying doing so by the time you complete the TAM Program." He pointed out that this statement might surprise us, since most people think of exercise as painful exertion, not as a feel-good enterprise. Or people will say they "exercise" if they occasionally swim, play golf or tennis, or take walks, so what's the big deal about incorporating exercise in a heart recovery program?

"Well, it *is* a big deal when it is scientifically programmed to meet the individual needs of each member of the group to accomplish the specific goal of improving one's heart functioning after an attack," Kevin stated. "Exercise in the TAM Program is a purposeful activity designed to produce a specific adaptation of the cardiovascular system. It's based on sound scientific principles, and when you exercise you'll be releasing the endorphins in your blood. Again, these substances kill pain and promote a high that makes exercise enjoyable."

The cardiovascular system (the heart and blood vessels) needs to be repaired after the damage done to it. Kevin told us that exercising in accordance with the individual exercise prescriptions made for each of us will contribute significantly to improving the way our hearts function. Research shows that aerobic exercise can:

- Lower high blood pressure
- Improve vascularization (blood flow)
- Normalize the heart rate
- Improve the heart's cardiac output (by normalizing the volume of blood expelled by the ventricles of the heart)
- Improve oxygen intake

- Lower the risk of another heart attack or stroke
- Increase HDL (good) cholesterol
- Fight obesity
- Help prevent osteoporosis
- Increase endorphins for feeling better
- Act as an antidepressant by improving one's self-esteem

In other words, aerobic exercise can help improve the quality of our life in general as well as our heart.

Differences exist between exercise in general and the aerobic program practiced at TAM. Aerobic exercise is any physical exercise that results in improved heart and lung functioning. To gain that improvement means using a regular program of exercise (not simply an occasional stroll in the park, swim or golf game) designed to accomplish the heart improvements listed above. Kevin worked with each of us to achieve this goal, but we each needed to take personal responsibility to establish a regular exercise routine—learned at TAM—and maintain that routine the rest of our lives. We needn't worry that we will be overworked and further endanger our heart, Kevin assured us. "We have evidence from our treadmill tests that we can predict what your safety margin is—how much exercise activity you can tolerate and how much you can improve that activity," he said.

In the question period, Kevin was asked about the difference between a typical rehabilitation program and the TAM Program. He explained, "In a typical rehabilitation program—a traditional one—exercise itself is the main goal. The big difference in the TAM Program is that exercise is considered a component of an entire program, not just exercise for its own sake. At TAM we combine the exercise program with nutrition, stress management, meditation and group support. It's a dovetail approach, since exercise itself can't be a cure-all. It's looking at exercise as an essential part of a healthy lifestyle that will maintain your heart in the best condition possible. Your self-image, your weight control, your stress and diet management—all these dovetail with the exercise program. To take an example, diet and exercise interact. Even if you take in the right amount of calories for weight control, those calories have to be of the right quality, since that affects your ability to exercise. Or, if there still is too much stress in your life, or you're feeling depressed, that will affect your ability to exercise and can have a harmful effect on your recovery. So, I have to be alert to all the components of the TAM Program, not just the exercise component, for me to help you get the maximum benefit from your exercise. That's what's great about the TAM Program: We function here as a coordinated team. Nothing makes us happier than seeing you improve the condition of your heart and the quality of your life."

Since I did not have a weight problem and walked my dogs regularly, even before my heart attack, I still had a "show-me" attitude toward Kevin's enthusiasm. My experience in the next eight weeks transformed me into a true believer.

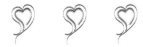

Alan Sadler, Stress Management Consultant: Managing Stress to Improve Your Heart

As Dr. Lawrence stated in his talk, managing stress through the TAM Program is key to improving one's heart condition. Alan Sadler, the specialist in stress management, had some very helpful thoughts about the subject. His talk proved to be an education in stress management. He taught Tai Chi and the Feldenkrais Method and how they can profoundly improve the physical and mental condition of heart patients. "Tai" means peacefulness, contentment, and restfulness, and "Chi" means energy. The combination means "peaceful energy."

Tai Chi consists of a series of defined movements that are dance-like and gentle. They are practiced over and over again with slow, deep breathing. "Practicing Tai Chi ten to twenty minutes a day, every day of the week on a permanent basis, will have extraordinarily positive effects for people with heart disease," he said. "Documented research shows that it's one of the best exercises for older adults and can improve heart functioning by reducing anxiety, fatigue, fear, tension and depression, among its many other benefits. Most important for heart disease patients is its ability to improve blood circulation and diminish hypertension."

Tai Chi is an exercise technique that originated in China some eight hundred years ago and has been taught in China for centuries. It's a basic part of Chinese health practice. Acupuncture and diet are also integrated in the Chinese conception of health improvement. In recent years, Tai Chi, just like acupuncture, has been gaining widespread acceptance in our country as an effective health-improvement measure.

Alan pointed out that Tai Chi is more than just exercise movement. It is included in Asian philosophy, which emphasizes that Tai Chi is a mind/body/spirit exercise. He explained:

> Tai Chi tries to train the whole person. It helps you discover the different parts of yourself and how they relate to your own self-image. It's a technique that looks beautiful and is very pleasing, which Western exercise can't duplicate. It's beneficial to the big muscles and circulation. Tai Chi contains power, but it's a soft, gentle power that doesn't jar the bones. It's also a form of meditation and has been referred to as "meditation in motion." You are really practicing mind/body harmony. In Tai Chi, your mind has to concentrate on the physical movements you make. You are always concentrating on your next move and not thinking about your problems. You are living in the present. In Chinese philosophy there is only "the now." That helps you build up a reservoir of peacefulness in your mind. Each day that you practice Tai Chi, you set aside a time building up this reservoir of peacefulness, where your energy is free, open and clear. It is when you block energy that you get sick. That's why the Chinese use acupuncture, as well as Tai Chi, to clear internal blockages.

This Chinese theory of health and wellness is now gaining respect in Western cultures. Believe it or not, this began to happen because when President Nixon went to China, he was cured of some illness by the application of acupuncture. When he returned he allowed acupuncture clinics to open, and the first acupuncture college was started right here in California in the sixties. Tai Chi and acupuncture work together when energy is severely blocked in a person.

Tai Chi focuses all of your attention on what is happening to you *now* because your mind has to concentrate on your movements and your breathing, so you don't have any room to worry about things. That's particularly beneficial to you as a heart patient, since it blocks out worrying about your condition and gives your heart more energy to heal. Your mind will feel quiet and open, and you are quite likely to feel you are floating and yet you are here on the ground, and with it come feelings of contentment. That's why Tai Chi is often called "meditation in motion" and is a great stress reliever. It gives you strength and gentleness.

Tai Chi is a great help to older people. In fact, it's one of the exercises you get better with the older you get. There recently was a woman in one of our groups who was in her eighties. But when you watched her performing Tai Chi, she looked twenty-five.

Alan also teaches the Feldenkrais Method. Both Feldenkrais and Tai Chi help you build a positive self-image and educate you to take charge of your life, to be a creator instead of feeling like a victim, which is so harmful to heart patients.

The Feldenkrais Method was originated by Moshe Feldenkrais, a physicist and engineer, who had been told by doctors he would never walk again after a severe physical accident. He refused to believe the prognosis and invented a method a few decades ago that enabled him to walk again. That method was found to help improve not only Dr. Feldenkrais's physical and emotional abilities, but also to help people who have had physical accidents, an illness, back problems or severe stress. Alan explained:

Feldenkrais developed a method of awareness through movement. Feldenkrais ties in with Tai Chi for heart patients in the sense that it helps you connect with the sensory, not the thinking, part of your being. You see yourself from the point of view of sensing your movements, how to move the big muscle group of your body, how to relax to reach the resistance point and not push through to the edge of resistance, then go back and move some other part of your body. The next thing you know, you get more flexible without stretching. So it's not like sports stretching, it's more using your brain to let go and create more possibilities of movement. Feldenkrais had a wonderful approach. He said, "You make the impossible possible, the possible easy, and the easy elegant." You'll learn the truth of this when I teach you the Feldenkrais movements.

Feldenkrais and Tai Chi both reinforce one's self-image. They give you the message that you can take charge of your life, that you can be a creator. They give you the ability as heart patients to create a positive self-image instead of a negative one. They both are tools you can use to improve your life by improving your heart condition, in conjunction with the other components of the TAM Program.

Since I was feeling like a wounded healer, the effect of Alan Sadler's talk was like receiving an endorphin high. It opened up new possibilities, particularly in its emphasis on "the now," when Alan remarked that Tai Chi is based on the philosophy that all we have in life is "now," the present. It affected me deeply, for that was so true of me as a heart patient. Treasure each day, enjoy oneself, focus on each day's possibilities, not disaster. My heart attack brought these feelings to the forefront of my consciousness. No fortune-telling about what could happen five years from now. The way I live each day will determine where I will be five years from now. The techniques Alan teaches could help me stop obsessing about the future, fearing the future, catastrophizing about the future. Now is all we have in life, whether we are sick or healthy. I heard the echo of *Now* in my mind and it sounded good.

Tana Ripley, R.N., Program Director of the TAM Program©: The Healthy Effect of Our Community-Based Program

Tana asserted that the lifestyle changes we would learn are necessary for improving our health, and that we can only become healthier if we practice them on a regular basis. She emphasized in her talk that the TAM Program was not an exercise program but an educational/experiential/behavior-modification program designed to create a healthy lifestyle for each and every member of the group. The education must be put into practice for the rest of our lives if we are to live longer by becoming healthier. I vividly recall her remarks on TAM as an integrated program: "Balance is absolutely key to the TAM Program," she said. "You can't just do part of the program. You can't just change your eating habits, just work on stress management or exercise, or just count on medication alone. It's a team effort of all these components working in harmony with each other that's the key to your gaining a healthier heart."

Tana continued:

The TAM Program is community based. Because of that, it can reinforce your ability to change your lifestyle more effectively than some other programs. For example, some reversal programs are "retreat programs." That is, you can leave home for a week, live in a hotel and then be exposed by their professional staffs to an education and practice program to improve your health. Everything is presented to you. You have no personal responsibility for preparing the dietary food, because their chefs do that. Here, on the other hand, we assist you in preparing proper foods, since we eat dinner here twice a week for the next six weeks. When you're on a retreat, it's easy to slough off or forget what you learned when you come home, because there is no follow-through support system. We were the first community-based program in the nation when we began six years ago. It's a way of fighting feelings of isolation that heart-disease patients like you might be experiencing. It's pretty typical to feel that way when you've had a heart attack. Feeling isolated is dangerous to your heart. The teamwork and the sense of community you will find at TAM will help you overcome that feeling. We're all here as part of a team, both the staff and you. We on the staff share in your happiness when you become healthier because that's our goal, too!

What Tana had said about TAM being a community-based program was very appealing to me. I had known from my work counseling divorced women that experiencing a feeling of isolation, which is also a feeling of hopelessness, can harm one's immune system and create great physical, as well as emotional, harm. Tana's advice about fighting isolation was a good reminder that I myself would now have to fight my own sense of isolation. I was now my own client.

Jan Keating, R.D.:
Food for a New Lifestyle

Jan explained to us that our diets have a great effect on our hearts:

Historically, one of the first observed connections to heart disease was the intake of fat in food to coronary artery disease and how excessive fat intake could contribute to heart attacks. Eating the wrong foods will disrupt your blood level, block your arteries, negatively affect your blood pressure, create obesity—all potentially life-threatening problems. On the other hand, a healthy diet can help stop heart disease from increasing, even help in reversing heart disease.

What all of you have had is a wake-up call that's saying you have to change your eating habits and your lifestyle to become healthier. They go together—the linkage between lifestyle and eating habits. If you have stress on the job, you'll eat on the run. Lunch becomes junk-food time. If you're sedentary, you'll spend the time eating all the delightful chocolates and high-cholesterol foods that will make you fat and ready for a heart attack. If you're unhappy, you are liable to use food as a substitute for love. But overeating will make you fat, not give you love. Your heart and your body will pay a terrible price when you do that.

Changing your lifestyle goes hand-in-hand with changing your eating habits, if you are to gain a healthier heart. That doesn't mean dieting to lose weight. Diets never work, because even when you lose the weight, you gain it right back. So I won't be talking to you about "diet." Instead, I'll be educating you about food choices. It's your decision about the food you choose to eat—how much and what kind—that will become beneficial or negative to your health. Food is either a weapon for or against you. It can create a better heart for you or another heart attack.

A diet's goal is a short-term loss of weight, not a change in lifestyle. That's why diets don't work. Diets have always been associated with dull, tasteless food. They have also meant giving up tasteful food and being hungry. It's associated with loss in life. All of you have had enough of a loss already. You'll certainly want food that's filling and tasty as well as being nutritional for your heart.

I have good news for all of you. There has been a revolution in low-fat food! You'll be educated in our program to be able to choose lots of very good foods that taste great. You'll also learn to read food labels very carefully. Because even though a food may be low in fat, it may be high in calories, so it's something to avoid. And even if a food is low in fat, it may be hydrogenated, which is saturated fat that harms the heart. Food with good nutritional value, like fruits and vege-tables, fish, lentils, beans, oatmeal and cracked-wheat cereals—which are very low in fat and have great fiber—are healthy for the heart. You'll find these foods filling as well as tasty. We even allow some meat in our food program, providing it's a very low-fat cut. Since fat adds taste to food, it's hard to give it up entirely. We don't do that in the TAM Program. A modest amount of unsaturated fat can be tolerated in a diet against heart disease.

Instead of diets, what we practice here at TAM is "food behavior awareness." That means choosing and eating your food mindfully to get the best help to your body and heart. People in general pay little or no attention to their behavior with food. If I ask, "Do you sit down or stand up when eating? What did you eat last night? How often do you snack and at what time? How often do you eat at the table or in front of the TV? What quantities do you eat? How many calories were in your last meal? Do you read the food labels?" most people don't know. These bad eating habits contribute to disease and illness. That is why at TAM we teach mindful eating. Remember, food can become your best friend for the rest of your life.

Jan noted an important difference between being a dietitian, which she is, and a nutritionist. "Anyone can become a nutritionist," she explained. "But a registered dietitian (R.D.) has a scientifically based background. A dietitian is a member of the American Dietetic Association, which has seventy-five thousand members who typically pursue continuing education credits and advanced degrees. A nutritionist is responsible to no one, so when you read something by a person who is called a nutritionist rather than an R.D. dietitian, take the information with a grain of salt. The problem with nutrition information is the credibility of the source. Be sure as a consumer to ask where the information comes from."

I found Jan's talk very informative, since I always

liked to bake and cook and experiment with new food combinations and eat new kinds of food. But I must admit I never used to read the tiny print on the labels that might inform me whether or not a product had hydrogenated or unsaturated fat or the number of calories. Even so, I thought I ate rather well, but I found I had much to learn. From now on, I would certainly pay attention to the difference between registered dietitians and nutritionists when I read food articles, which I like to do.

Laura Arnold, R.N.: Positive Reinforcement Through a Group-Support System

Laura shared with us the reason she is so personally enthusiastic about the TAM Program:

What the TAM Program provides for people with heart disease is a wonderful opportunity to change lifestyles so they can have a healthier, happier life with a better-functioning heart.

In my seventeen years of working as a nurse in critical care units prior to my experience with the TAM Program. We would advise heart patients to watch their diet, stop smoking and get some exercise. That would be all we had time for, or all the patients could absorb in their traumatized condition. But it often didn't work well. I kept seeing people come back, sometimes with more heart problems a year or so after they had an attack. We clearly didn't have all the answers.

New scientific data has shown that you need more than dietary and exercise support. You need stress-management techniques also. That's because your emotions can affect your heart as much as diet and exercise, as Alan Sadler explained to you. The great thing about the TAM Program is that it incorporates these stress-reducing techniques, which traditional rehab programs don't do.

In addition, we have a group-sharing support system. You'll find it very enlightening and tension-reducing when you join it, because you'll discover that the other people in it have many of the same concerns you have. You'll feel comfortable sharing the same kind of issues they have. You may find it to be a great problem-solving experience. We do things in a group because being in a group makes for a stronger bond. You get positive reinforcement from each other, which makes your adherence to the program more likely. In fact, at least 80 percent of the people who have been through the TAM Program continue in their daily life to incorporate some of the techniques they've learned.

Listening to Laura intensified my yearning and need for a connection with a community. She reinforced what Tana Ripley said. In my work as a psychotherapist, I need to be neutral, to be "above the battle" in dealing with my clients if I am to help them. But now I needed to be helped, I needed a support system. This was a new experience that stirred up a lot of mixed feelings. I had to fight my feeling that my needing group support was a sign of weakness, that I was a "failure" because of my attack. I had always thought of myself as a strong person. I would have to learn—as I did in the next eight weeks—that you can be strong by asking for and accepting support when you need it. In fact, it's a sign of weakness and fear when you don't seek out and ask for such support when your health requires it.

Dr. Mark Wexman, Medical Director of the TAM Program©: A Doctor's Personal Commitment

Dr. Wexman pointed out that an enormous number of men and women—up to seven hundred thousand—die each year of cardiac-related causes like stroke, hypertension, diabetes or other vascular diseases. In fact, it's become a Western-culture norm for people to die of this problem.

He said, "People in general, however, are confused about the nature of heart disease and need to be educated to the fact that the vast majority of heart disease is coronary heart disease—or atherosclerosis, the hardening of the arteries. But there are also valvular heart disease and rheumatic heart disease, which used to be very common years ago but now are mostly preventable. Coronary heart disease, which the TAM Program treats, is overwhelmingly the most common kind in America, 80 percent to 90 percent in fact. This is not true worldwide, because it's a Western-culture disease, and as more western European countries adopt our American lifestyle—our stress, our bad eating habits, our lack of exercise, our overweight problems—they too are at risk of an enormous prevalence of coronary heart disease."

In the question period, Dr. Wexman was asked why he became a surgeon. He answered:

On a purely professional side, I had an intuitive understanding of cardiac physiology that drew me to it. I liked it, I understood it, it seemed to make sense to me. I also had an ability to relate to the personalities of cardiac patients. My father died a sudden death. My father had Alzheimer's. He was a teacher who always did for others and not much for himself. He seemed to be physically well, but had memory problems and was diagnosed in his late fifties with Alzheimer's. My father died at age sixty-seven. He had been feeling fairly well when he went out for a walk on the day he died. He came back to the house while my mother was out shopping. My father collapsed at home, but the nurse who was with him did CPR and revived him. My father, who hadn't talked in eighteen months, said, "Don't call 911, I'm feeling much better now—just get me a blanket, I'm a little cold." And he carried on this conversation I now know verbatim. And then he died. Now, I cannot explain my father's improvement in cognitive mental function based on oxygen and blood deprivation that we know occurs in a period of sudden death; in a scientific, physiological way I don't get it. In a mystery-of-medicine way, I look at this as my father's soul being closer to the surface. My father's soul did not have Alzheimer's, but my father's brain may have. When he had his near-death experience and was passing on, his soul was accessible somehow. I know there is a history of sudden death in my family and that was a big deal, and that's why I am involved in cardiology. I know that my work matters and I know I can make a difference, and that makes it worthwhile for me to pursue.

I was moved by his passionate statement, his personal commitment to saving people's lives. This commitment, in fact, was the defining characteristic of the entire Cardiology Associates' staff that spoke to us that weekend. This was a professional group dedicated to serving people, not a money-making machine.

Another aspect of his talk that stays with me three years after I joined the program was his statement about the objective of the TAM Program. He said, "This program is not what you deprive yourself of, it's about what you substitute in terms of other healthful things that I think will improve the quality of your life more than what you are giving up decreases it."

When I heard him say this, I hoped it would be true. As I write this three years later, his prediction is no longer merely a hope: It is simply the truth of my life today.

6

Moving Ahead

MAJOR EXTERNAL AND INTERNAL CORONARY ARTERIES

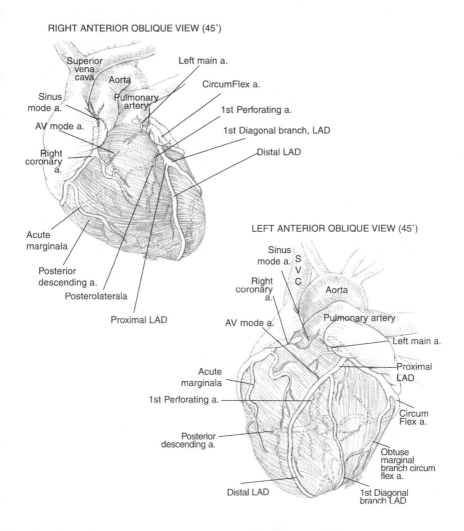

RIGHT ANTERIOR OBLIQUE VIEW (45°)

Superior vena cava
Aorta
Left main a.
CircumFlex a.
Sinus mode a.
Pulmonary artery
1st Perforating a.
AV mode a.
1st Diagonal branch, LAD
Right coronary a.
Distal LAD
Acute marginala
Posterior descending a.
Posterolaterala
Proximal LAD

LEFT ANTERIOR OBLIQUE VIEW (45°)

Sinus mode a.
S V C
Right coronary a.
Aorta
AV mode a.
Pulmonary artery
Left main a.
Acute marginala
Proximal LAD
1st Perforating a.
Circum Flex a.
Posterior descending a.
Obtuse marginal branch circum flex a.
Distal LAD
1st Diagonal branch LAD

I must take personal responsibility to change my lifestyle if I am to live. . . . That was the red-light message repeatedly sent to all of us in the group by the TAM staff at the marathon meeting. The repetition was necessary because change is never easy, particularly when it means changing the way you live your life. Even when you know that advice is true, good intentions to practice it can fall by the wayside, like New Year's resolutions usually do.

I would have to fight against using phony excuses to slacken off from adhering diligently to the TAM Program. (I still have to fight this tendency today, long after I have left the program.) But I always win this battle, because remembering my near-fatal heart attack tells me that diligently pursuing the program means living, and slackening off means dying. My choice is to live, so I adhere to the program rigorously, illness or unavoidable time-consuming situations being the only exceptions to this rule.

What had so impressed me about the introductory TAM Program talks was the staff's emphasis on what we heart-attack patients could control to reverse our heart disease. Surprisingly, uncontrollable factors that can cause heart disease and accelerate new heart problems after a heart operation are few in number. These uncontrollable factors are heredity (a genetic predisposition in one's family or origin to have attacks at an early age); age (the older one gets, the greater the possibility—in women particularly—to have a heart attack); and gender (postmenopausal women have more heart attacks than men).

These uncontrollable elements, however, are not as significant as they were once believed to be. In what I believe is the best book ever written on the aging process (*Successful Aging,* by John W. Rowe, M.D., and Robert Kahn, Ph.D., Random House, 1998), the authors state that while heredity is important in promoting disease, it is less important than one's lifestyle. TAM also takes this position and proves it by its success rate in preventing and reversing heart attacks in women and men who have an inherited tendency toward heart disease. Neither is there the need to feel victimized by your age or gender, since changes in lifestyle are also more important in preventing, causing or reversing heart disease. So what is inevitable in life—heredity, age, gender—doesn't mean inevitable illness, nor that death is around the corner.

A heart-disease patient like myself needs all possible hope, since hopelessness about surviving the disease can result in death as a self-fulfilling prophecy. As Dr. Lawrence pointed out, there is scientific justification for believing that emotions can have either a positive or negative effect on one's heart condition. Hopeful emotions are positive health reinforcers; hearing from the TAM staff that this assertion was scientifically valid was a powerful motivator for me to adopt a positive attitude about the possibility that I could reverse my heart disease.

Being assured that controllable risk factors are more significant than uncontrollable ones (such as age, genetics and gender) gave me great hope. The TAM Program identified those toxic components of my lifestyle that I had the personal power to eliminate, with the assistance of the TAM Program and staff:

Smoking. The worst killer of them all! The AMA Web site revealed that a woman who smokes is two to six times more likely to have a heart attack than a woman nonsmoker. Over half of all heart attacks in middle-aged women are due to smoking. My heart attack was one example.

There is no safe level of smoking. Even smoking ten cigarettes a day doubles the risk of heart attack. Smoking damages heart arterial walls, creates high blood pressure, and causes blood clots that lead to strokes and heart attacks. As if that's not horrid enough, the carbon monoxide generated by smoking reduces the amount of oxygen needed by the heart to function properly. And don't forget about the increased risk of lung cancer.

I had worried that smoking at least a pack a day for twenty-five years before my heart attack would prevent my heart from healing, even if I stopped smoking. But Dr. Sklar reassured me that once I stopped, no matter how long I had smoked, my risk of having another heart attack would drop by at least 50 percent. Within two weeks after I stopped smoking, the carbon monoxide level in my blood would be reduced to normal, restoring the oxygen smoking had taken away from my heart.

So my heart disease would begin to reverse itself, but only if I took personal responsibility never to smoke again in my lifetime. Secondary smoke can also have a heart-disease/cancer-producing effect, even if you personally have never smoked. So quitting smoking and avoiding secondary smoke offer the added plus of helping your heart and preventing lung cancer.

Hypertension (high blood pressure) is an excessive amount of force exerted by blood against the walls of the arteries. The higher your blood pressure, the greater the damage to your arteries, which can cause great strains on your heart and weaken it. Hypertension is also the major cause of stroke. It's called "the silent killer" and is present when your blood pressure is 140/90 or higher ("140" when your heart, which is a pump, contracts, and "90" when your heart is relaxed). High blood pressure is a silent killer because most women are unaware of its importance or even that they have it, even though screening in a doctor's office is easily available. Over 50 percent of people with high blood pressure are unaware of it. The good news is that blood pressure can be brought down to normal levels without risk.

High LDL Cholesterol Levels. LDL is the "bad" cholesterol. The "good" kind is HDL cholesterol. Cholesterol is a fatty substance that helps form various tissues in the body. The "bad," LDL, cholesterol is one of the major causes of plaque in arterial walls, and high amounts of it can trigger heart attacks. On the other hand, "good" HDL cholesterol destroys the fat that LDL cholesterol circulates in the blood, strengthening heart arteries rather than weakening them. Diet and exercise can increase good cholesterol. Good foods are foods rich in fiber, fruits and vegetables. Bad-cholesterol foods are animal-fat foods—meat and dairy products.

Overweight and Obesity. The fatter you are, the greater the possibility of a heart attack. Postmenopausal women in particular are prone to putting on extra pounds. Each excess pound is a stepping stone on the road toward a mortuary. Being overweight can cause a weakened heart, a build-up of bad cholesterol in the arteries, hypertension or diabetes. Exercise and diet can arrest this criminal assault on your body and heart. A fast, moderate exercise combined with a healthy low-calorie diet can reduce a woman's risk of heart disease by 50 percent or can begin to reverse the disease in those who already have it.

A Very Sedentary Lifestyle. Since the heart is a muscle that needs energy to pump normally, it requires exercise to function efficiently. A sedentary lifestyle creates conditions for heart disease, diabetes, stroke, low self-image and attacks against the immune system. These risks can be diminished by including more physical activity in your life. I learned that 60 percent of women participate in no regular exercise activity. I suspect that postmenopausal women are even more likely to avoid exercising. But then comes the wake-up call of the presence of a disease, like my heart attack, which demands that we make exercise an essential part of our lives.

Estrogen Deficiency. Menopause is a time of estrogen depletion. Prior to menopause, the hormone estrogen is a major protector against heart disease for women. Estrogen offers protection against blockage in blood vessels. When menopause depletes estrogen below the premenopausal, heart-protecting level, women can become more susceptible to heart attacks. Insufficient estrogen causes LDL cholesterol—the bad kind—to create additional plaque formations in heart arteries, resulting in blockages that can cause a heart attack or stroke.

New findings indicate estrogen levels after menopause can indeed be raised, which can significantly lower the risk of a first or subsequent heart attack. The fear that "estrogen replacement therapy," as this is called, might have the side effect of producing cancer has been found to be excessive. A balance of estrogen and the hormone progesterone in the postmenopausal years can effectively diminish any cancer side effect, while also preventing further heart disease.

Stress Overloads. The kinds of stress Dr. Lawrence talked about can be lethal: Anger or hostility, for example, makes the heart beat abnormally fast, tenses muscles and creates hypertension. It's a menu made for a heart attack. The emphasis of the TAM Program on relaxation and meditation techniques designed to reduce this kind of stress seemed to me to be one of the most promising and hopeful aspects of the program.

Drugs and Alcohol. I list these two separately simply because in our society alcohol has been socially acceptable and not thought of as a drug. Yet the reality is that alcohol is the drug that is more dangerous to the health of the men and women in our country than *all* the other prominent "recreational" drugs (cocaine, marijuana, heroin) combined. All of these drugs can cause a heart attack or stroke, but excessive alcohol intake is the major contributor to this disease. Cancer, liver disease, strokes and diabetes are but a few of the consequences of alcoholism. Drug addictions, including smoking, are difficult to break. But the choice is always a personal one for someone with a heart-disease problem: Break the habit or die.

Combined Diseases. As we've noted, postmenopausal women suffer heart attacks much more frequently than younger women. Since women heart-attack victims are usually older than their male counterparts (in their fifties, sixties and seventies), they may also have additional age-related diseases, such as diabetes, breast cancer or arthritis, making many women more vulnerable than men to a second heart attack. The combination of diseases also makes recovery harder. A woman with diabetes, for example, will be two to three or more times more likely to sustain a heart attack than one without diabetes. What's more, she would also be at greater risk afterwards, because diabetes cancels out the positive effects of estrogen on her heart.

Thanks to modern medicine, the diseases a woman may have in addition to heart disease can usually be managed through careful monitoring so as to minimize their possible negative effects on the heart.

MY PERSONAL INVENTORY

How did my heart condition relate to the controllable and uncontrollable factors listed above? After attending the TAM marathon, I took a personal inventory, starting with the factors beyond my control:

- **Age.** Mid-fifties.
- **Genetic Inheritance.** No record of heart disease in my family background. No record, either, of diabetes, a foremost cause of heart disease.
- **Gender.** Female, therefore more susceptible to heart disease since entering my postmenopausal years.

I then itemized the controllable factors:

- **Smoking.** The overwhelming cause of my heart attack was smoking a pack a day for twenty-five years.
- **Hypertension (high blood pressure).** I did show a genetic tendency toward high blood pressure; family relatives had it. I knew my blood pressure was high (180 over 100) when it should have been below 140 over 80. I would sometimes work to lower it in earlier years, but never worked hard enough to prevent it from returning.
- **Cholesterol.** Excessively high levels of cholesterol (that is, over 200, with the "bad" cholesterol measuring over 130 and the "good" cholesterol less than 35) is dangerous to the heart, because it can contribute to hardening of the arteries. At the time of my heart attack, my cholesterol level measured 250, with my "good" cholesterol down

to 25, which helped create the excessive plaque that resulted in damaging my heart.

I had inherited a genetic tendency from my family background to have a high cholesterol level, as well as high blood pressure. However, recent scientific evidence offered convincing proof that changes in my diet and exercise lifestyle could bring my cholesterol level down to or below 200, in spite of my dangerous genetic tendency.

- **Exercise.** Aerobics would have meant daily, consistent exercise to stimulate my heart and blood circulation, something I never did. I would swim occasionally and walk my two Maltese dogs daily, but never increase my heart rate to a workout level. I had plenty of room for improvement here.

- **Weight.** It's never been a problem for me (I'm lucky, I guess!). I'm five feet, eight inches, and my weight has never exceeded five pounds above my normal weight of 150. At the time of my heart attack, I weighed 155 pounds.

- **Diet.** Before my heart attack, my diet tended to contain a mixture of lots of fruits and vegetables (good!). But I also liked hamburgers, hot dogs, cold meats, lamb shanks, fried potatoes with lots of salt, bacon (a favorite), nonskim milk, and ice cream and chocolate candies for dessert. I indulged in lots of oil for frying and cheeses for eating. And pasta (I'm half Italian), which I loved to prepare with lots of butter and meat sauces. So the diet that Jan Keating suggested was much different from my regular diet of the past few years, which was loaded with calories and saturated fat. Since I don't eat a lot, my diet had less effect on my weight than if I had been a clean-everything-off-the-plate eater.

- **Drugs.** I never tried marijuana, cocaine, heroin or any other trendy drug. I quit drinking alcohol ten years ago; even though I never drank more than two or three glasses of wine in an evening, it still seemed excessive to me. There was a genetic tendency toward alcoholism in my family on my mother's side—her father died of alcoholism, but she never drank. I decided a decade ago that "none" is the best drink of all, and never regretted taking that action.

But I was addicted to the worst drug habit of all: smoking!

In summing up the positives and negatives of my lifestyle inventory, the negatives unfortunately outweighed the positives. On the positive side, I was not addicted to any drug (except nicotine); I was not overweight, give or take a few pounds; I did exercise a bit, if sporadically; my food intake was on the modest side, for I never gorged myself; I did not have any other disease. . . . In fact, my body was in good shape except for the debilitating effect of my heart disease. My attitude toward life had always been upbeat, even though I had more down feelings after my heart attack.

This positive list of my lifestyle factors prior to my heart attack seemed rather modest when I contrasted them with the negative elements I would have to change:

- **Smoking.** I would have to eliminate smoking from my life, now and forevermore. I had not smoked since my heart attack six weeks previously, but still felt in the past few weeks, as I was beginning to heal, a strong desire to return to the habit. *No way!* This was going to be a severe internal struggle. It's one thing intellectually to know that the return to smoking will kill me, but it's quite another story to fight the craving to inhale the cigarette smoke that I had been so physically and emotionally addicted to for those twenty-five years of my life.

- **Hypertension.** Since I had had the experience in previous years of being able to lower my blood pressure, I felt confident that I could change this aspect of my lifestyle permanently. I needed no greater incentive to do so than my heart attack.
- **Cholesterol.** Lowering my cholesterol to a normal level would be a real challenge for me, since I never made the effort to do so before. Jan Keating, the dietitian in the TAM Program, reassured me that even with a genetic tendency such as mine it was perfectly possible with a proper diet and aerobic exercise to bring my cholesterol level down to normal, and for it to remain there permanently. I was determined to live up to Nancy's prognosis.
- **Exercise Habits.** I would have to learn and practice aerobic exercising. I still had only the vaguest idea of what that meant. Would it be hard or easy to incorporate this exercise as part of my new lifestyle? I felt some trepidation because of my ignorance. But Kevin, the exercise physiologist, would be my coach. He seemed warm and very competent, so why worry in advance? Maybe I'll even like it!

- **Stress Overload.** Whatever severe stress I felt in my life before, like the deaths of my parents and the divorce from my first husband, was matched by my present state of mind. I was under even more intense stress because it was present in my life every moment of my waking hours and also disrupted my sleep. What will happen next to me? How can I plan for the future? Will I be able to continue my practice as a psychological counselor? Should I tell my patients I had a heart attack? Would I frighten them away if I did? Will I be a basket case, needing to rely on my husband and my children as if I were a needy little child begging for help? Will I be a shadow of my former self, wasting away in fear and despair?

My mind kept jumping around like a wild monkey as these thoughts ricocheted inside me. I seemed to have an endless reservoir of anxiety. Will it ever stop? The TAM staff had reassured me that once I began to take personal charge of my life by adhering to their program, the stress overload would begin to disappear. If the light at the end of the tunnel was to be the beginning of a new lifestyle for me that would overcome all of the negative elements in my pre-heart-attack lifestyle, that would be fine. But what if the light at the end of the tunnel was the light of an oncoming train, a new heart attack—over and out permanently? These mixed feelings could only be resolved by making the effort to change my lifestyle in accordance with the TAM Program. *Keep the faith in new possibilities, fight the fears within me,* I told myself. *Keep the faith.*

7

I Practice My New Lifestyle

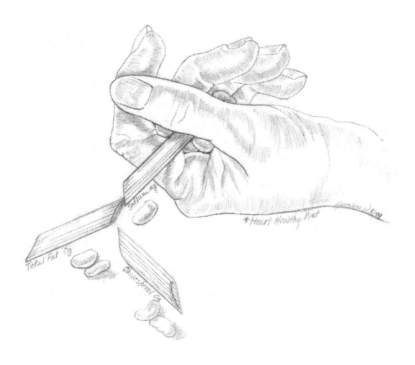

I Stop Smoking Forever

Six weeks after my heart attack, I hadn't smoked a single cigarette. It didn't take much willpower then to refrain from smoking, for I was too sick and too scared to even think about cigarettes. But by the time I attended the TAM marathon, a yearning to puff a cigarette again emerged, and I fought it immediately. All I had to do was remember what Dr. Sklar told me in the hospital: "Never take even a single cigarette again if you want to live!"

All of my fears that I would have a terribly difficult time giving up smoking were based on my two previous halfhearted attempts, eight and four years ago, to stop. They failed after a two- or three-day try. I felt then I was hopelessly addicted. I had also heard so many stories from clients I had counseled about how they failed too, which seemed to justify my failure.

But a happy surprise was in store for me. I did not find it that difficult to stop permanently and never again experience any craving to light up again. Four months were all it took for me to eliminate even the urge to smoke again! My craving had vanished and never came back. My husband, Mel, was amazed how quickly I overcame my smoking habit. He had stopped smoking seventeen years ago and said it took him three years before he ended his craving (and he had gained fifteen pounds by substituting eating for smoking). He told me he frankly thought I would never give up smoking. "You knew you should give it up, but you always had excuses not to," he remembered. "You would say, 'I'm smoking a lighter cigarette now,' or 'This brand has less nicotine,' or 'This new filter makes the smoke purer!'" I pointed out to Mel that there is all the difference in the world between trying to stop smoking on one's own, without having an illness (like he had done it) and being told, like I was, that smoking even one more cigarette would pave the road to my death. I couldn't fudge even once if I wanted to live.

I can smile now at my resistances before I reached my goal of kicking the smoking habit. When Dr. Sklar told me in the hospital that I would have to give up smoking forever, my initial response was, "Do I have to?" I thought then that I loved my cigarettes; when I ran out of them I used to immediately run to a store to replenish my supply. I would think of how I enjoyed a smoke just before I went to bed. If I woke up in the middle of the night, I would smoke another one. Inhaling my cigarette used to give me a bit of a high. And smoke from other people's cigarettes gave me a pleasant feeling. I eliminated these "pleasures" of smoking by substituting new, healthy pleasures that I learned about in the TAM Program. I began to lose my craving for cigarettes when I did my aerobic exercises. These exercises made me center my attention on my physical activity, leaving me no time to think about smoking. I used to say to myself, "A workout a day keeps cigarette-smoking away." Aerobics give me an endorphin high that was better than any high cigarettes ever gave me. Tai Chi was also wonderful in reinforcing my determination to end my habit.

The TAM group-support meetings made me feel I was not alone in trying to break my smoking habit. Others in the group had the same kind of experiences I had. We fought tobacco together.

At home, I developed new techniques to conquer my smoking habit. Gum was a great cure! During those four months I bought what seemed like mountains of all flavors of sugarless gum—peppermint, spearmint, cinnamon and even bubble gum. I substituted these wonderful flavors in place of cigarettes. I would hold five pieces of gum in my hand, sometimes even ten, so whenever the slightest craving for a cigarette showed up, I'd pop another piece in my mouth—spearmint was my favorite—and my cigarette craving would go away.

I also ate a lot of low-fat foods I could chew during the day—celery, carrots, raw peas, and red and green peppers—to compensate for not smoking. And I found new food combinations in the TAM diet program that made me forget smoking.

I felt that I really wasn't giving up something, I was getting something better. That something better was a new lifestyle from the TAM Program that made me focus on the healthy, positive things that matter in life. Then it happened suddenly—four months after my heart attack, on the ninth of May—I woke up and my craving for cigarettes had totally disappeared! The yearning had stopped! I had new things going for me in place of smoking, so I would be a fool if I ever reached again for a cigarette.

I am writing this three years after I stopped smoking. Secondhand smoke, which can also be a killer, is something I also totally avoid. I try to leave a room where smoking is occurring. I'm not a prude, I'm just being realistic. If other people still want to smoke, it's their choice, but how sad. Whenever I see a woman light up a cigarette in the street, I have an urge to say to her, "Honey, you better throw that thing away, because it's going to kill you and you don't even have a clue that it will. You'll think it will happen to everybody else, but not to you. It will, though. Yes, it will."

Ironically, my heart attack made me stop smoking—very quickly! I can think of much better ways to kick smoking than having a heart attack. But in my case, a near-death heart problem has saved me from an inevitable death from smoking.

I Monitor My Medication

The prompting from my doctor concerning medication was the same as the one he gave me for smoking. I must take six different tablets once a day, plus an aspirin tablet, and keep nitroglycerine tablets on hand in case I ever have an oxygen intake problem. I must take four tablets after breakfast and two after dinner every single day of my life until the doctor tells me to change. Without monitoring my medication and taking it as prescribed, the alternative would be devastating: I would die.

I needed no more education or coaching to convince me to take my medication appropriately, for the echo of what Dr. Sklar told me remains with me every day. Three years after he gave me my prescriptions, they are an essential part of my daily life—not a delightful part, but a necessary part. When I open my medicine cabinet in the morning, I see those bottles standing like soldiers guarding my health. They protect my blood pressure and cholesterol levels, lowering both of them to normal levels. Today, both levels *are* normal, thanks to the medicines in collaboration with the rest of the components of the TAM Program.

I learned from the TAM Program that each heart-attack survivor receives an individual medical prescription. Some persons experience side effects, even from aspirin, so what I was given for my specific problems of high blood pressure and high cholesterol would differ in kind and amount from others who may have different problems. It's always the right thing to rely on a personal evaluation from your doctor and disregard any conventional wisdom suggestions. I was indeed fortunate, because once my medication was fine-tuned to appropriate amounts, I have experienced no disturbing side effects from any medicine in the past three years. I am convinced that careful monitoring by myself and my doctor of appropriate intake levels is absolutely necessary. I can still remember my horrible experience right after I came home from the hospital before we were monitoring carefully.

Monitoring and adhering to my medication regimen was easy. But when it came to aerobic exercise, Tai Chi, Feldenkrais and diet, I needed all the TAM education and coaching I could get. After the TAM marathon, I eagerly looked forward to the twice-a-week TAM Program, which was to last eight weeks.

Every Tuesday and Thursday I would show up for the TAM Program, which lasted from 5:15 P.M. to 9:30 P.M., and included the following:

A. Aerobic exercise was first, with a warm-up at the beginning and a cool-down at the end.
B. Second was Tai Chi and Feldenkrais movements.
C. Third was a group-sharing experience that began with five to ten minutes of sedentary, silent meditation.
D. Fourth was dinner, including TAM staff lectures.

I Experience
Aerobic Exercise—And I Like It

When I saw all that mechanical equipment in the exercise room at Cardiology Associates on that first day of my program, I felt anxious and intimidated. *What on earth am I doing here?* was my first impression. *These look like men's things, not for women.* The last regular exercise course I ever had was in high school, which seemed like centuries ago. Some swimming, some basketball, some softball . . . that was all. I would look at some of the girls in that gym class with disapproval. They were the muscle-bound ones who took exercise very seriously. They seemed to be forever lifting weights. They looked so unfeminine to me. I gathered the impression that too much exercise was harmful to my femininity.

Most of the men in the TAM group seemed to take these aerobic instruments in their stride, like they were familiar acquaintances. But Kevin Roberts, the aerobics instructor, had said at the TAM marathon that aerobics meant special physical exercise that would increase my heart and lung efficiency, which I urgently needed, so I reconciled myself to learning to use the equipment and overcoming my fear of it.

But I really had nothing to fear (like any exertion on my part would cause another heart attack). Kevin was a superb coach who monitored everyone in the group and tailored the amount and pace of exercise to never exceed each person's healthy limitation point. We would be protected from any dangerous overexertion.

The first day I was introduced to all of the aerobic equipment: a treadmill, a Stairmaster, a stationary bike (Cyberbike) and a UBE (for strengthening the arms). I was assured that each person had his or her own individual exercise goals to attain. I learned how to start the machines and how to make them function properly. Kevin started me off very slowly and increased my speed the more confident I became. I used each machine for ten minutes, all with the objective of strengthening my heart.

As the weeks rolled by, I began to enjoy my growing expertise and the endorphin highs the exercise gave me. My target rates increased and I became stronger. The exercise had a positive effect on my self-esteem. I remembered that the TAM Program emphasized that each member needed to take as much personal responsibility for improving his or her heart as possible. Each exercise session would begin by recording my weight and my pulse (which I would do myself) and my blood pressure (taken by a rehabilitation adviser). A warm-up period ensued, followed by exercise on the machines. After using all the machines, there would be a cool-down period. Each member was responsible for monitoring his or her pulse rate after each activity. This kind of personal monitoring made me feel less like a victim and more like a person in charge of my own life, taking responsibility for making it better. I felt like I was a partner in the TAM Program. Kevin carefully evaluated our records to determine how well we were functioning and how we could stretch ourselves to function better. Every time I met my target I felt proud of my achievement. I would then prepare to achieve an increased target rate, and I would feel a real sense of personal power when I made the new rate.

I have continued to participate in an exercise program for one hour every Monday, Wednesday and Friday morning, ever since my TAM Program ended. Today my heart rate is normal. I completely changed my attitude towards exercise. I no longer consider it a necessary evil; instead, I see it as a positive, permanent lifestyle addition that is saving my life. I have become so expert with the aerobic machines that even some men who are newcomers to aerobic exercising ask me how to operate them. I'm pleased to give them the benefit of my expertise!

I long ago lost my fear that I would become a muscle-bound, unfeminine woman by exercising regularly. I'm still slender and tall, and feel stronger, but in no way am I muscle-bound. Women of my generation really need to eliminate the old-fashioned notion that fitness programs are a male prerogative. We could use as role models the younger generation of women who incorporate those programs as part of their everyday life. The exciting emergence of the American women's world-championship soccer team is testimony to the reality that all forms of exercise are prerogatives of women as well as men. It would be unfeminine to believe otherwise.

Tai Chi and Feldenkrais©
Come into My Life

With Tai Chi, it was love at first sight. I felt so immediately when I saw Alan Sadler at the first session demonstrate the flowing, elegant movements of Tai Chi as the model we as a group would follow.

Tai Chi was a monitored group exercise. The women in the group seemed to take to it immediately, given that Tai Chi had closely resembled ballet movements. On the other hand, the men in the group were more awkward in the beginning, like Dr. Jason Lawrence, who thought initially it was "too feminine," and therefore felt uncomfortable and a little embarrassed practicing the Tai Chi movements. But the more the men practiced it over the next eight weeks, they became firm believers in Tai Chi as a stress reducer and physical tune-up exercise. Indeed, as Alan had stated in his talk at the TAM marathon, Tai Chi was "meditation in movement." The exercise forced me, as well as everyone else in the group, to center my attention on the present, on "now." The movements we were performing forced us to concentrate solely on the present movement and the next one we would have to make. The movements we made were ritualized. We would repeat the same movements over and over again during the eight-week sessions. I became very adept in my Tai Chi movements over time (I had always loved dancing and this was so similar).

I indeed experienced a sense of peace—a letting-go of the past and of worrying about the future—as I practiced this lovely art form and exercise. I also enjoyed the group experience. All eleven of us practiced together, and I felt bonded with the group as we connected spiritually toward the common goal of healing ourselves.

The same feeling came as we practiced the Feldenkrais method of physical movements, which occurred after Tai Chi. We also did this in unison. While Tai Chi was a standing exercise, Feldenkrais involved lying on the floor mat, with Alan supervising our movements. The movements were also ritualistic, to be repeated over and over again during the eight weeks. Feldenkrais was designed to strengthen the spine and develop new brain pathways that would enhance our body movements. Many group members commented on how much their spine improved and how back pains that they had lived with for many years were eliminated because of Feldenkrais. I never had back-pain problems, but I found Feldenkrais very helpful in reducing the built-up tension in my mind and body.

Each member of the group had his or her own special enthusiasm. Obviously, the people who had suffered spinal or back-pain problems were more delighted with Feldenkrais than other people. My favorite was Tai Chi. Tai Chi was—and still is—my first exercise/meditation love. I'm delighted to see Tai Chi gaining greater acceptance nationally, on television programs for one, where it is most visually impressive. I have seen programs that show groups of hundreds of people over age sixty-five practicing Tai Chi in unison. On the other hand, I have seen people in their twenties also enjoying the experience. It's truly a universal exercise and meditation art form.

After the Feldenkrais exercise, our group would sit on chairs in a circle and silently meditate for five to ten minutes. Tai Chi, Feldenkrais, and silent, sedentary meditation were related to one another. They all were designed to reduce the stress and tension that kept pervading our lives as a consequence of our heart attacks and of our previous lifetime habits. Meditation through exercise—combined with traditional seated meditation—powerfully cleansed me of the stress overloads I brought to each meeting.

Laura Arnold would usually direct the silent meditation exercise. She first suggested we hold hands with each other while she outlined how we were to meditate effectively. She set the stage for us to relax, to visualize a peaceful state for ourselves. She told us that we personally were in charge of our own meditation, which would relax our body and calm our minds. She read to us in our first session a statement from the National Institutes of Health, the most prestigious governmental health organization in the United States, that clarified the meditation technique we were to use. It read: "The meditator makes a concentrated effort to focus on a single thought—peace, for instance; or a physical experience, such as breathing; or a sound (repeating a word or mantra, such as 'one'). The aim is to still the mind's busyness—its inclination to mull over the thousand demands and details of daily life."

Laura then suggested we stop holding hands (which emphasized our group connectedness) and close our eyes and begin to silently meditate for five minutes, each person to concentrate on a single thought or sound of his or her own choosing.

I had been familiar with this kind of meditation for a number of years previous to my heart attack, but never practiced it on a regular basis. Although I had found it very valuable, I thought I was too pressured to find daily time for it. Now it would be incorporated in my daily life, something I welcomed rather than resisted. In my personal five-minute meditation, I would usually choose to concentrate on the word "peace." The result was remarkably similar to my experience with Tai Chi— a feeling of relaxation and restfulness, a letting-go of time and place (sometimes these five minutes, with my eyes closed, seemed like two seconds, other times like five hours!). My heart and breathing rates would improve as my stress overload reduced.

For almost all others in the group, this kind of meditation was something new and foreign. I noticed many of the men had a difficult time in the early sessions of just sitting still. In this kind of meditation the injunction is, "Don't just do something, sit there instead!" and men usually feel that "not doing anything" is a guilty waste of time. They felt vulnerable in having to close their eyes, as if someone would take advantage of them while they couldn't see. However, by the time the eight weeks were over, many of the men discovered that they were strengthened by meditating and would also practice it at home. They told me they had accomplished more in meditating and sitting still for five minutes each day than they thought possible, particularly in lowering the severe stress they were feeling, not only from their heart attacks, but also from their jobs. Other men, who were in the minority, felt the meditation was a waste of time and said they were unable to center their mind on a single thought or activity. These people had had a mindset from the beginning that meditation was nonsense, and that attitude turned into a self-fulfilling prophecy.

The women, on the other hand, had no such resistance as the men. They all were open to this new experience, and at the end of the eight-week program they expressed how valuable meditation had been for them and stated they would include it in their daily lives. In general, the fears of the men in the group when they were given new things to do, like Tai Chi or sedentary meditation, seemed to generate a knee-jerk anxiety reaction in them. It was as if anything they didn't know was beyond their control, which made them feel helpless. So new approaches to exercise were seen more as a threat than a promise to better their lives, while the women had no such fears. "After all," one woman told me, "that's why we're here, to learn how to improve our hearts. The new things we learn truly help me."

I really enjoyed the seamless flow of the exercise training we had: First a warm-up (we would warm up to the tunes of peppy jazz music), then the exercise on the aerobic machines, then Tai Chi and Feldenkrais, and, finally, sedentary meditation. At the end of each session I always felt enlivened. My mind and body seemed to be telling me, "Your cholesterol level is becoming more normal and so is your hypertension. Keep with it, Pat." I began to really feel I was taking charge of my health rather than feeling victimized by my illness.

I Discover I Like My New Low-Fat Diet

From 5:00 P.M. to 6:30 P.M. on Tuesday and Thursday nights, the group had a low-fat meal in the Cardiology Associates' dining room. Everything we ate was made in accordance with the principles of the TAM Program: complete elimination of saturated fats ("hydrogenated" oil is a saturated fat), but all fruits and vegetables and fish were allowed. Low-fat soups, bread made with unsaturated oil, and desserts such as low-fat sherbet, yogurt and fat-free ice cream were also allowed. I learned, to my surprise, that the TAM diet allowed for a modest amount of meat intake— low-fat cuts of meat like beef and skinless broiled chicken and baked turkey breasts.

In the beginning, I focused on what I had to give up in the way of food, rather than what I would gain from my new low-fat diet. My old diet was on the high-fat side. I had never paid any attention to reading the fine print on the labels that identified the fat intake of a product as saturated (hydrogenated) or unsaturated. True, I was a very modest eater; I was always satisfied with a small intake of food. That was in my favor. I never liked fatty meats, which was also a plus. But, oh! the butter, the cheeses, the mayonnaise, the hot dogs, the hamburgers, the ice cream, the chocolate bars, the luscious cakes I used to make would now disappear forever from my life. It was as if a part of me was dying and I was mourning the loss of all the goodies that always had been a part of my daily meals and snacks. It took me some weeks on the new low-fat diet to convince me to say good-riddance to my old diet (which I now called "the killer"). My taste buds began to change, and I found the new diet arrangement actually tasty as well as healthy. I must say I wouldn't have subscribed to the new diet voluntarily if I hadn't had a heart attack and was told: "Eat the new way, or have another heart attack!" But my taste buds changed to enjoy the new diet. I could even drink skim milk instead of fat-saturated milk: the skim milk began to taste better than I thought it could. I recently tried an experiment. I tasted some of the whole milk I once had with every meal and then tasted the organic skim milk right after it. The skim milk tasted fine in my mouth, the whole milk tasted awful! Three years of drinking only organic skim milk had turned my taste buds around, proving you can accustom yourself to any food when you have the willpower to do so.

I moved—with less resistance than I expected—from a perception of food deprivation to new diet acceptance after the first few weeks on the TAM diet. I noticed I didn't feel deprived when I had excellent substitutes for my previous, excessively fat diet. In place of my old fatty ice cream, I began to enjoy low-fat yogurt and low-fat chocolate sherbet. (Chocolate is my favorite flavor!). I always liked fish, so I had many dinners of fillet of sole, steamed salmon, shrimp and crab. Squeezed lemons made a perfect substitute for the mayonnaise I had always liked. I loved whole-wheat bread, so that was no change, except that I made sure it was made with low fat of the unsaturated kind. Vegetables and fruit salads I had always loved. In my new diet I could still eat them, making sure I used a low-fat dressing or lemon juice or vinegar on my vegetable salad, and no dressing on my fruit salad. Once a week I would eat some slices of baked turkey breast (baked with no fat) or a broiled chicken breast. This would be supplemented with fruits and vegetables. As for dessert, gone were the apple and lemon meringue pies and chocolate cakes that had been favorite parts of my past life. Dessert now became low-fat yogurt or sherbet or fat-free ice cream. A low amount of unsaturated fat was allowed in each day's meal. For me, it was 20 percent fat, for others it could be less, since TAM doctors and dietitians tailored the fat amount to each individual's needs. The range was 10 percent to 20 percent, with 20 percent being the highest amount allowed.

My new diet provided much variety once I learned that it was a friend rather than an enemy. One of the fun things we did at our TAM dinners was to exchange new discoveries of food we could eat. Every Tuesday dinner was a potluck dinner. Each group member was supposed to bring a low-fat dish for all to share, along with a recipe. We were given free choice to bring what we wanted, without demanding it be an entree or dessert or appetizer. It has always surprised me that on every Tuesday the eleven people in the group brought a sufficient variety of foods so that appetizers, an entree and dessert were always present! Was the universe telling us something?

Each of us brought some dish to be proud of. I was so happy that the borscht I made with nonfat chicken broth and tomato sauce with onions was so well-received. My other successes were my baked turkey breast and low-fat pasta.

On Thursday nights, the Cardiology Associates chef made the meal. Sam was a superb chef who taught us a lot about how to learn to cook low-fat style. Most of his recipes were delicious. He taught us tricks like substituting applesauce for shortening in chocolate cake. While we were eating dinner we would have a lecture by some member of the Cardiology staff. Sometimes it would be the dietitian, Jan Keating, and sometimes it would be one of the doctors, or Kevin Roberts educating us about exercise. Dinner was never dull. We were able to ask all kinds of questions after the lectures. For the first time in my life, I was aware of the calories listed on the package and the kind of fat in the packaged product I would buy. My calorie amount was set at a target level where I would not gain any weight, but I would actually be able to lose a few pounds (I was five pounds overweight at the start of the TAM Program and lost these pounds by the time it ended). Since each person in the group had a different weight problem, the calorie target levels would vary widely from person to person, based on what the doctors and dietitians considered appropriate.

We were allowed a "guilty pleasure" on occasion. After a month, I could savor and eat a chocolate ice-cream cone, or buy a chocolate cake or an apple or lemon meringue pie and allow myself to be nostalgic. I never used meat as a guilty pleasure. Somehow, the memory of my hot dog and hamburger eating days had vanished.

I have continued with my diet and am still enjoying it. In the magazines and newspapers, I am always alert to articles with new low-fat diet recipes that seem worth trying. All of these elements have made my new lifestyle diet an achievement instead of a deprivation.

I have not yet mentioned the group-sharing experience that occurred each Tuesday and Thursday. I am leaving that for the next chapter, which will deal with the psychological impact of my heart disease and subsequent surgery and recovery. It is important enough to deserve a chapter in its own right, for in understanding my own shattering emotional response to my heart attack and its subsequent effect on my ability to take personal charge of healing my heart, I was able to understand the emotional reactions of the ten other members of the group in similar circumstances. Our combined struggle to achieve self-renewal mirrors a world in which managing illness is a lifetime necessity, a world millions of men and women inhabit.

8

The Mourning Process: The Pathway to My Self-Renewal

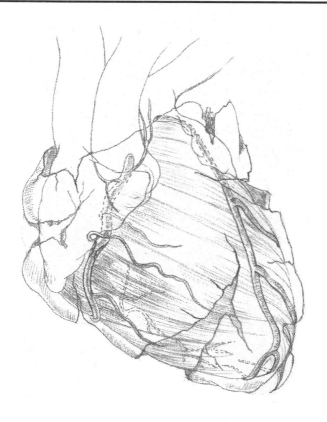

The TAM Program gave me a specific means to reverse my heart disease. My body was telling me it was working: the combination of appropriate medication, exercise, diet, and meditation and group sharing was reducing the plaque in my arteries, strengthening my body's resistance to infectious diseases (which could precipitate another heart attack), and making me feel less of a victim and more of a person who could make positive things happen in the face of an overwhelming disaster.

And disaster it was. There is no sense in denying the critical nature of my illness. I had been a breath away from death, and that enormous fact had a profound effect on my sense of self. In those first weeks after I went home from the hospital, prior to my joining the TAM Program, I would look in the mirror and what I saw wasn't the familiar "me." The mirror returned an image of a weak, drained woman with pale skin and haunted eyes that were drenched with fear of the present and fear of the future (if I had a future). I felt as if I had aged ten years.

Had I remained in this state of mind, I would not be

alive and able to write this book today. The mind and the body work together—and the mind can destroy the body, or help to heal it. If you feel you are a victim of forces beyond your control (and that is what a heart attack initially feels like), you may contrive to act like a victim and give up fighting for your life.

I felt that way for a short time. I can still recall that early stage after my heart attack when I tried to avoid looking at myself in the mirror, because what I saw seemed like a horror story. At that time, I felt I was living a distance from my pre-heart-attack self, the rock-solid self that was always there to do my bidding. That "rock" seemed to have turned to sand. It was just like the 1989 San Francisco earthquake I had lived through, when my house shook like a ship on a wild sea as the ground beneath my feet started to give way. I felt then the sharp fear of not being able to count on what I could always count on, the very ground beneath my feet. That ground now proved untrustworthy; it could swallow me up instead of supporting my ability to continue with my life. I felt that way in those uncertain early days after my heart surgery. My body, like the ground beneath my feet in that earthquake, had betrayed me and become my enemy. The world was now a very scary place with no one to trust, since I could no longer trust my own body to do my bidding. My heart was beating out the words, "You can't count on me."

Other aspects of my behavior at that time also frightened and disoriented me. Why did I feel so sad twenty-four hours of the day? Why did I break down and cry so frequently? Why was I so super-sensitive? If a friend told me a sad story, I cried. If a movie or TV program had a sad ending, I cried. One day I stopped my car for a blind person crossing the street in the pedestrian zone, and as she fumbled her way along, tears flooded my eyes. Of course, she and I were the same, we were both fumbling along not knowing where we were headed. And for no reason at all, when I was driving alone in my car, tears filled my eyes. I was even afraid to turn on the car radio because news reports of crashes and deaths could make me cry.

What was happening to me that caused such disarray? I never used to cry. In fact, when my mother died, my relatives were surprised I didn't cry at her funeral. It took one whole year before I could really cry out, indeed shriek out, my internal pain over my mother's death. When it came to crying, I was always a stoic, but now I was a puddle of tears.

In the midst of my sadness, anger that seemed to come from nowhere would explode within me. I was brought to self-awareness about my anger in a humbling experience I had while driving downtown. In front of me was a car with a rather old lady behind the wheel who was driving slowly; she was going ten miles an hour in a twenty-five-mile-per-hour zone. I heard a burst of sudden anger come from my mouth. "Darn it," I shouted to no one in my car, "why doesn't that old lady drive faster? How dare she creak along." I honked my horn impatiently, but there was no response; her car kept to its very slow speed. Then I saw her left light flashing, and she turned into a funeral parlor where somber men and women were arriving.

How ashamed I felt! That old lady could have been the wife or relative of the person who had died. I thought about my rising anger against her and my irrational outburst and felt like a fool. I had always prided myself on my compassion and coolness when driving, not letting any tensions on the road control me. Yet here I was being "out of sync" with my former self.

From that incident, I became aware that I was feeling irritable over any little thing, forgetting where I placed my pocketbook, "losing" my keys at home. I sometimes frightened myself by believing I lost my purse—my identity was lost—when it was safely in the place I had left it. I, who had always been so well organized, was becoming a chaotic mess, helpless and disoriented.

From Despair to Enlightenment

I wrote in chapter 3 about all the positive help I received from my husband, Mel; my sister, Peg; and my two daughters, Vickie and Karen, and how it reinforced my will to live and prevail over my heart disease. It was their help, combined with my own motivation to triumph over my heart disease, that made me join the TAM Program. However, at that same time, there was "another woman within me" warring against my hopeful attitude, a despairing and fearful woman. The hopeful "me" won the upper hand, but not without a struggle. In order to conquer my despair, I had to find out why I was acting in such irrational ways, so I could eliminate those feelings of being a helpless victim, feelings that could make me self-destruct in spite of my desire to live.

It was while this emotional conflict was still raging within me that I joined the TAM Program. Through my belonging in the TAM group's sharing and support meetings that took place for a minimum of one hour twice a week, I found the key to why I was experiencing self-defeating emotions along with my positive emotions.

I used the word *belonging* in that last sentence because that is what it felt like—not "joining" the group, not " being with" the group, not "attending" the group, but *belonging* in the group. A we're-all-in-this-together spirit made the eleven members more than just eleven separate individuals. All of us were bonded together by the same narrow escape from the abyss of death, and we needed each other's strength to return us whole to the physical world that was almost taken away from us. That was the symbolic reason for all of us joining hands at the beginning of each session and then silently meditating for a few minutes before sharing our individual concerns. We needed no words to know that we were spiritually connected to each other in our need for validation, that our damaged hearts did not make us damaged persons. However, this feeling of connectedness did not emerge immediately. It was first a hidden presence, only to blossom after two or three sessions when we came to know each other better. Then our concerns about each other's welfare opened up. Each of us brought new low-fat recipes or talked about a new food discovery that was tasty and could be included in our diets; we shared articles from newspapers and magazines about developments in heart-disease research; we brought books and video tapes, and recommended lectures and TV documentaries about our condition; we even met later on at each other's homes for potluck dinners—all acts of kindness and caring. Then and only then did our personal feelings surface.

I was not only an integral member of the group, I also was an observer of the group—two persons in one—for I was a group counselor myself. Part of my own professional expertise was being the group leader of men and women who needed help in their marriage or divorce problems. I knew that members of a group are initially guarded, uncertain or ashamed to share their personal experience with strangers. They feel they may be judged and found wanting as "good" persons. Soon enough, after a few sessions, a group becomes a secure place to share oneself at deep personal levels in order to find the help and support needed to solve problems. This is exactly what happened to our TAM group. All of us were very guarded in the beginning, myself included. It turned out that the cause of this guarded, don't-come-too-close-to-me quality we exhibited was depression. We felt our self-image was damaged, that our body had betrayed us. We feared that our diminished ability to function as we formerly had would cause our family, friends and acquaintances to no longer love us or like us. Our guardedness also covered our internalized anger. We were angry over the loss of our former ability to function as we had at home, work and play.

I observed all of this in the first two sessions of the group meetings. Suddenly it all came together—the reason for the wild swings in behavior that I described above and that I brought to the group sessions. I connected my own depressed feelings with those that I'd felt when my mother died and when I was going through the traumatic divorce from my first husband. Both were terrible losses, and now I was experiencing another terrible loss, the loss of my old self-image: the image of strong, healthy Pat, the Pat who could take long walks, play an aggressive game of tennis, stay up late at parties, climb hills, carry heavy bags of groceries from the supermarket, and worry only about doing my counseling work as effectively as possible because I loved helping people. Gone! Gone! Gone! My feeling of loss, now that I was in touch with it, was overwhelming. To accept help, instead of giving it, was repugnant to me. That would be a "Pat" I never was. Yet here I was seeking help, asking for it.

Once I became aware that I was experiencing profound loss, the pieces of the puzzle about why I had been feeling and behaving in such a contradictory way, in which hope and despair contended with each other, fit together. Whenever someone experiences an overwhelming loss, the immune system sets in operation a "mourning process" to enable that person to regain his or her health. In my work as a psychotherapist, I had helped many men and women regain their health, and a new positive sense of themselves, when they were severely depressed over the loss of a loved one or over a divorce (which is the death of a relationship). I would help them move through the mourning process, which is the need of both body and mind, emotions and behavior, to come to terms with a relationship no longer present and a way of life that had depended on that relationship. The death of a spouse and the breakup of a long-term marriage require the need to mourn in order to make way for one's self-renewal. New adjustments in our behavior must be created if we are to regain our ability to create positive things in our life. A divorced person mourns the loss of his or her identity as a married person and learns to become self-sufficient as a single person; a widow or widower mourns the loss of a spouse and renews herself or himself as a separate individual who now incorporates the dead spouse as a spirit rather than a physical presence in her or his life. To accomplish these objectives, a person must live through a mourning process, a series of stages each involving different emotions and behaviors that enable a person to recover from the loss.

My feelings of loss were no different from those I'd felt over my mother's death and my divorce. Yet I had gone through the mourning process in those two instances and had emerged a better person. My mother is always a spiritual presence within me now. Her values, her compassion for the underprivileged, her participation in volunteering to better her community, her kind and sensitive parenting, her passion for self-knowledge, her fight against injustices—I carry these values within me, and when I act on them it is my mother, as well as myself, acting on them. Out of the anguish I felt over her death, my mother made me a better person. I have mentioned how my divorce, which at the time seemed like the end of the world to me, became instead a new beginning that transformed me from a housewife into a psychotherapist.

I personally had experienced all the stages of the mourning process in order to reach these goals. And the first stage always involved my feeling depressed! The symptoms of depression were now present with my heart disease: feeling irritable, helpless, fatigued, worthless, guilty, restless, and the fear of not being able to function in the world as I once did, which would make me frequently cry. As I indicated in chapter 3, denial of the seriousness of my heart attack and then the shock of its seriousness arose within me shortly after I had returned home from the hospital. That shock and denial are part and parcel of the depression experience.

If I was depressed at the time of my first group-sharing visit, then what about the other ten people in the group? Were they experiencing the same sense of devastation that I was? The clues were all there at the first session: everybody seemed guarded at first. After identifying themselves by name, they would say little. Small talk dominated talk about the exercise they were doing, the new low-fat food they were eating, the new recipes they discovered in their favorite magazine. It was like there was an elephant sitting in that room with us that everyone was afraid to notice. That elephant was our heart disease and the emotions it caused. Our magical thinking was: if we don't talk about it, our heart disease will go away. But that elephant refused to budge. Fear and bleak uncertainty remained with us all through that first session.

When I left that first session I felt curiously elated. That group session had given me a great gift: the gift of self-knowledge that I was involved in the mourning process arising from my heart attack—and that everyone else in the group was similarly involved. It may sound strange that I felt "elated" at my discovery that all of us were in the initial stage of the mourning process, depression being a major factor in that first stage of mourning. (I was elated because being involved in the mourning process meant I was healing instead of dying.)

I learned from the TAM staff that excessive crying is typical of both men and women shortly after heart surgery, as are sadness and depression. They also told me that depression is an acute, usually short-lived response; that, indeed, it is part of the healing process most patients undergo as they begin to take greater personal charge of their lives in the TAM Program. An angioplasty such as I underwent, or a bypass operation, is an invasive assault on the body, and crying is the body's way of trying to heal.

This fact was certainly evident in my group as the weeks went by. Each of us was getting physically stronger through aerobic exercise; our fear over the future was diminishing as we discovered we could actually take charge of improving our health; the stress-reduction program of meditating in motion (Tai Chi and Feldenkrais) and sedentary silent meditation was reinforcing our immune systems. Our changed diets made us feel healthier and lose weight. We were responsible, in association with the TAM staff, for these positive results. We felt more powerful; less victimized; more in charge of new lifestyles that would enable us to manage our heart disease, reverse it and live constructive lives without worrying every moment if another heart attack was just around the corner.

The Four Stages of the Healing Process of Mourning

The mourning process in heart-disease patients typically works through four stages, as follows:

I. The "Why Me?" Stage

First comes the shock and denial of experiencing a heart attack. (Remember, I only had "a severe case of indigestion" and kept denying to the paramedics that I had suffered a heart attack.) To save one's life, an immediate angioplasty or heart bypass surgery is frequently indicated. My angioplasty took place very quickly after I arrived at the emergency room, because the longer the wait, the greater the damage to the heart. Getting to a hospital within three hours after an attack can save your life. A longer wait, even six or seven hours, could mean death.

In the early weeks of recovery, symptoms of depression predominate. Like a nightmare visitation, the soul cries out, "Why me? What have I done to deserve this? It's so unfair!"

II. The "If Only" Stage

If you are in a constructive environment like the TAM Program, the initial "why me?" shock diminishes in direct proportion to the changes in your lifestyle and the group support you receive from relatives and friends as well as from professionals.

The mourning process in Stage II shifts from denial and depression to recriminations about the past. Yes, you have heart disease which you no longer deny but, rather, acknowledge as a poignant reality. Sadness, grief and regret define this stage. Your old way of life has disappeared, but a new way has yet to emerge. You experience yearnings for what was lost and despair over never being able to recapture the past.

III. The "Letting Go" Stage

Paradoxically, hope begins to emerge out of the despair experienced in Stage II. Kierkegaard once observed that in Christian terminology death is the expression of the greatest spiritual despair. "The cure," he said, "is to die—to die from"; that is, to die from despair and the illusion that you can recapture and remake the past. ("If only I never took up smoking. What a fool I was. My life would be so different now!" was the regret I had to give up). Stage III enables you to sever the illusion that you can change the past. That means "dying from" that illusion, which provides the ground for you to move forward in the present, rather than remain trapped in past regrets.

IV. The "Self-Renewal" Stage

In this final stage, all of the wide-ranging feelings and contradictory behaviors you lived through in the previous three stages diminish, so that they become distant memories of your past, rather than regrets that continue to overwhelm you and immobilize your present life. You begin to feel capable of making more positive things happen in your life, that life still holds new possibilities for you, instead of inevitable disasters. Self-flagellation turns into self-acceptance based on who you are now, not on what you once were.

In many ways, you are healthier now by adhering to a program like the TAM Program. Your self-renewal is based on your changed lifestyle, a physical change involving weight reduction, plaque reduction, improved heart circulation, and a strengthened body. Self-renewal also comes from a new, more spiritual outlook that focuses on living fully in the present and appreciating the gift of life, which becomes more precious as you eliminate unnecessary stress in your daily existence, the stress that turns life into an obstacle course instead of an enlightening journey.

The Goal: A New Sense of Yourself

As one progresses from each of the first three stages of the mourning process, a sense of termination is present. This feeling provides the framework for self-renewal in the fourth stage. However, there is no ending of Stage IV, the self-renewal stage. Self-renewal is a lifetime journey. Indeed, we will have to pay attention to our medication, our exercise, our diet and our meditation for the rest of our lives. But standing on this solid ground enables us to move continually in new, more fulfilling directions.

In the three years since my heart attack I have seen such renewal take place in many of the former members of my TAM group. I share some of their stories below:

- A lawyer whose heart attack was generated to a considerable extent by overwork and intense stress arising from dealing solely with personal-injury cases changed his career to cyberspace law. He works at home and makes as much money working four days a week as he once did working five, and has found the time to learn to play the piano, a lifelong dream.
- A divorced woman who lived in isolation prior to her heart attack has reached out and become involved in Mended Hearts, a national organization of heart-disease patients who meet regularly to reinforce their ability to renew their lives. She has found the new friends she formerly despaired of ever finding.
- An owner of a small company posts a sign on his office door every day that says, "Do Not

Disturb—I'm meditating for the next fifteen minutes!" He has become a kinder, more sensitive boss, and has created a warmer, cooperative atmosphere for himself and his workforce. This approach has diminished excessive turnover and increased productivity in his company.

- A woman whose marriage was tearing apart before her heart attack recognized that she indeed did love her husband, and he her, more than they both had realized. They renewed their twenty-three-year marriage by going to a marriage counselor after she left the TAM Program and are now feeling closer to each other than they had in many years.

- A man told the TAM group he had been terribly depressed, but medication combined with the TAM activities helped him overcome his condition, which enabled him subsequently to divorce his wife. Both of them had long acknowledged their incompatibility, and repeated efforts had failed to diminish their unhappiness. Neither of them had the courage to end their mutually destructive relationship. He said, "During the last eight years of our nineteen-year marriage, it felt to me like the torture of ten thousand cuts, as the Chinese saying has it. It was only after my triple-bypass operation that I realized how stupid it was to continue the torture of my marriage. My heart attack was a wake-up call for me to make the most of time, and my divorce now has allowed me to do exactly that." His divorce also turned out to be a positive experience for his ex-wife.

- A woman who underwent an angioplasty had been alienated from her son and her daughter for six years. They were grownups who lived on the East Coast, three thousand miles away from her, and had two children each. Her heart attack triggered an entire reevaluation of her relationships with her children. The arguments that alienated her from them now seemed trivial in light of her heart attack, and she yearned to see the grandchildren she had never seen. She wrote her son and daughter long, thoughtful letters, apologizing for past hurts and misconceptions and expressing the desire to see them again. Her children were also ready to renew their relationship and responded positively to her letter and offered to pay her way to visit them. She accepted the offer, and now she has the loving connection with her children and grandchildren she thought was never possible. "I never realized that life gives us a second chance for happiness. My only regret is that it took my heart attack for me to get that message," she told me.

- A widowed woman whose husband had died five years before she underwent bypass surgery came out of her cocoon as a result of TAM group support. She now derives great satisfaction from working with an organization that helps homeless people secure food, clothing and shelter. "These are people much more in need of help than I am. I think my husband George is looking down and approving what I am doing," she told me.

- A thirty-eight-year-old man discovered he could survive and actually become healthier in many ways after his quadruple-bypass operation. He came from a family that had a genetic tendency to die young, some as young as age thirty. He once thought that would be his inevitable fate. Now he no longer believes this. The doctor at TAM assured him he has a long life ahead. The operation was successful and he was in good physical condition. He feels he can plan for the future and has decided to marry the person he loves. He had avoided doing so out of fear he might die a year or two after marriage, which would be a horrible thing to inflict on his loved one. Now he feels excited about marriage and children becoming a part of his future.

Other people I contacted experienced no surface changes, but the mourning process effected powerful changes in their attitudes toward work, marriage and children. They became kinder and more attentive to their family and delighted in pleasing them rather than complaining about their behavior. They experienced their burdens at work as feather-light rather than as a hundred-pound knapsack, as one of them described it to me. "Nothing" had changed for them, but in a deeper spiritual sense, "everything" had changed.

Some men and women became "stuck" in the first, second or third stage of the mourning process and never moved onto the self-renewal stage. When I called one member of our group, a businessman, two years after he attended the TAM Program to find out how he was doing, I received a curt answer: "I don't think about that anymore. All I wanted to do was return to my job in better condition and I did that." He then said, "I'm busy, I have to go now." It was as if I had threatened him by reminding him of his heart disease. He obviously was still stuck in the first stage of the mourning process, when denial of one's serious condition and avoidance of deep-seated fear of the future have the upper hand. (I later learned that he continues to regard his heart attack as a past problem and took up smoking a pack of cigarettes a day, a habit he had broken when he attended the TAM Program. I keep my fingers crossed about his welfare.)

Other group members were stuck in different stages of the mourning process. One woman always looked sad and said very little. It was almost as if she weren't a member of the group. Three years later, when I spoke to her over the phone, she still sounded sad. This time, however, she revealed why: While she was recovering from her angioplasty, she learned that her eighty-five-year-old father decided to undergo bypass surgery for congestive heart failure, from which he had been suffering for half a dozen years. "He told me that it was better to risk surgery than live in agony with his disease," she said. "I was worried silly when I was in the group, because his surgery was scheduled for that time. One week after the group ended I heard he had died on the operating table. His heart had been too damaged for him to survive. And a year later, my mother died of emphysema. She was eighty-two and smoked until she died. With my own heart attack, I felt like it was too much. But I survived with the help of my three grown sons and some dear friends. It's taken time, but I now feel I'll be okay."

After talking with her, I felt confident she was becoming "unstuck" and would ultimately move to the self-renewal stage.

Such examples of the mourning process in operation reveal there is no set time for mourning to occur.

Each person experiences it at his or her own pace. The more a person understands the healing function of the mourning process and how it can be utilized to strengthen one's will to establish a new lifestyle that will reverse one's heart disease, the sooner the stage is set for self-renewal. And if one recognizes that one is "stuck" in an earlier stage of the mourning process, psychological counseling can help end the feeling of hopelessness and empower a person to move forward. The people who take full advantage of the healing potential of the mourning process are those women and men who adhere strictly to changing their lifestyle. The elements of change are both physical and emotional and in one form or another are always combined in a manner similar to the TAM Program. It means a permanent dedication to a changed lifestyle. Without that permanent change, self-renewal will always be an illusion rather than a reality.

Mourning is a process that allows one to heal over time, and affords one the opportunity to take charge of his or her life positively after the trauma of a heart attack or the discovery that one has heart disease. Taking advantage of that opportunity transforms living into the promise of a full life by prevailing over one's heart disease rather than succumbing to it.

What About Sex?

Sex and heart disease . . . a myth prevails that heart disease and intercourse are an oil-and-water mix. The belief that sexual exertion for those who have a heart problem will trigger another heart attack—or death—

is still widely accepted by the general public as well as by heart patients. The good news is that modern scientific findings disprove this myth. We who have heart disease need all the good news we can get!

I have not written about sex in relation to heart disease earlier in this book because it is not a top priority when a person has a heart attack and surgery. Recovery is the top priority, getting healthy, remaining alive—these are the priority issues that needed attending to in our group. But as our health improved, the question of sex and our ability to regain our capacity for the kind of sexual gratification we experienced prior to our heart attack and surgery did begin to surface. It surfaced very hesitantly in the group. All the men and women seemed to be waiting for the person next to them to discuss the topic. For we all saw sex as a "problem" (I must confess I, too, had that concern), an activity that may be impaired because of our heart disease.

One member of the group was brave enough to say, "Let's find out what Dr. Sklar has to say about sex!" You could almost hear a universal sigh of relief. "That's a great idea" was the unanimous consensus.

When Dr. Sklar was asked to attend the next session of the TAM group and enlighten us on this subject, he said he would be delighted to do so. His lecture was wonderfully reassuring. Here is the "heart" of what he told us:

> Is there a risk in having sex after a heart attack? Well, the risk is no different than any other exercise of similar vigor! We doctors believe that you should get back to normal sexual activities within a reasonably short time

after a coronary event, just like you should get back to any other exercise. The reason you should get back to it is that a big part of having heart disease is its psychosocial aspect. If you become isolated from your partner, if you change the pattern of your life, if you change your sleep patterns and your exercise patterns and your sex patterns, you will end up unhappy. Your psyche will become altered, and that is not a good thing. Communication is good, closeness is good and if sex is part of that closeness, then it's good for you. If you have had a heart attack, how long should you stop intercourse? Maybe weeks, not months. Sex with your spouse or partner is not a coronary risk. People in stable relationships really do well.

We now felt we had permission to talk about our concerns about how sex would once again fit in our lives. We had so many questions that began to emerge:

- Would my sexual drive return?
- Now that my sexual drive has returned, will I have another heart attack if I initiate sex?
- My operation has given me an ugly scar; will my spouse or partner reject me?
- How can I satisfy my partner when I feel so unattractive?

All of these concerns were based on fear that we would be labeled second-class citizens if our sexual selves were impaired. In particular, our loved ones might now think of us as being unworthy of their love.

Sex has been so overemphasized in our society that we have been brainwashed to believe that our sexual performance is a major definition of our self-esteem. And sex, according to our cultural conditioning, means intercourse. We have the view expressed by that sexual authority, President Clinton, who stated, "If you say two people are having a sexual relationship, most people believe that includes intercourse."

Of course, this is absurd. President Clinton was able to say he never had sex with Monica Lewinsky because he "only" had oral sex, which was performed solely by Ms. Lewinsky, hence no "sexual relationship." He proved, unwittingly, by his own actions with Ms. Lewinsky, that a sexual relationship has a far wider range of connotations than coitus. A coitus-centered definition of sex defines only one function of sex (and not necessarily an essential one). This fact has been validated time and again in public-opinion polls—in direct contradiction to the excessive emphasis on sex-as-intercourse, or as a prelude to intercourse—in ubiquitous movie and television shows (without such sex, you don't amount to much as a person is the subliminal message of the media). The public-opinion polls tell a different story: When people are asked what is the most important thing in life for them, they always respond with "a loving, caring relationship" as their first answer. On a list of ten of the most important things in life, "sex" usually ranks fifth or sixth, and "money" around seventh or eighth.

I know from my own experience as a psychotherapist for the past twenty years that this is true. Sex is an expression of a relationship, not its definition. I have counseled couples who endure miserable relationships, but who claim their sex life (many daily orgasms) is great. Yet they feel unloved and alienated from each other. After their nightly arguments and four-letter-word accusations, they usually have sex. Their "great sex" in the form of intercourse and multiple orgasms is used as a tranquilizer and as a denial of their estrangement from each other. Each of them feels unloved by the other, and sexual intercourse does nothing to assuage those feelings. Sexual intercourse is their Band-Aid.

On the other hand, I have known couples who feel loved and soulfully connected with each other and for whom intercourse once or twice a month is quite satisfactory. There are also gay and lesbian couples involved in long-term monogamous relationships in which the variations on physical intercourse are of little or no consequence to their relationship. Their love for each other is their paramount concern. It is the loss of intimacy, the erosion of closeness, that causes heterosexual and homosexual couples to seek my counseling, and that central concern may have little to do with the quality and frequency of sexual intercourse.

Indeed, I have seen couples for whom sexual intercourse is irrelevant. The man may be impotent because of an illness and the wife does not see this as a deprivation. Their love for each other is very real and they seek out alternative means of physical gratification (mutual oral sex, hugging, cuddling, kissing). But they tell me their feeling of being loved, their belief that love also means caring for each other in sickness as well as health—caring as a gratuitous act, rather than as an onerous obligation—means for them a sexual closeness without intercourse. The novelist Alix Kates Shulman wrote a beautiful phrase about caring of this type: "In the scales of fulfillment, devotion may sometimes outweigh freedom."

As these examples demonstrate, sex is an individual issue: What's enjoyable for one person or couple may be unacceptable to another. As for sexual "performance," number comparisons are meaningless: Couples may derive satisfaction from intercourse once a month or once a day or never, yet all of these relationships may be equally valid if the couples themselves find their particular arrangement satisfactory.

When I am asked what's the best perspective from which to evaluate sex and sexuality, I like to quote the philosopher Ortega y Gasset, who observed, "Nine-tenths of that which is attributed to sexuality is the work of our magnificent ability to imagine, which is no longer an instinct, but exactly the opposite: a creation." In other words, nine-tenths of sex is in the head instead of the bed.

Mel and I have always felt that when we write a book together, when we counsel clients together, when we plan new projects together, when we help each other renew our courage in the face of adversity—all this is a form of making love, of validating each other as whole persons, sexuality included.

To be loved for who you are, to want the best for each other as individuals and as a couple—this is the desire of most adults in our society. And where a relationship has been a loving one prior to being struck by heart disease, that relationship will remain rock solid after returning from a hospital. As one husband told his wife who had a bypass operation, "I didn't marry you because you didn't have a chest scar, I married you because I loved you as a person and still do. Your chest scar is not you. It's something I never notice!"

Even persons like myself, who like to believe that we are not influenced by the media, may feel initially that maybe we are less worthy of love after surgery. Such is the brainwashing power of the media. It's best to talk about your feelings with your spouse or partner. I did this with Mel and cleared away my downgrading of myself. "Stop judging yourself; I love you with or without angioplasty," was his response to my concern, and he gave me a hug.

Some of the women and men in our group found it difficult to discuss sexual concerns with their partners when the group sessions ended. They carried those concerns like black clouds over their heads, fearing their partners might be rejecting them. They were trying to read their partner's mind and had no right to believe, in advance, that their partner was rejecting them because of their heart attack. I heard from some of these couples in the past year who shared these issues with me. They said they had solved it by going to a good marriage counselor where they felt safe to communicate their fear of rejection because of their low self-esteem. Their relationship improved (and so did their sexual feelings) once they discovered in counseling that their partners did not love them less. Those who continued to believe they were unattractive because of their heart disease but never told their partners about their feelings and resisted the idea of going to a good counselor found that their relationship became very unhappy and in some instances resulted in separation or divorce.

And then there were some in the group who needed only reassurance from Dr. Sklar that regular, active sex was not harmful. They remained as sexually active after their heart attack as they were before. And they enjoyed it as much as they previously had. Their fear that their sex urge would never return turned out to be false.

When couples come to me for counseling about their sexual problems, I like to give them a favorite passage of mine, written by the great novelist D. H. Lawrence, which places sex in what I believe is its proper place in any relationship:

For sex, to me, means the whole of the relationship between man and woman that lasts a lifetime, and of which sex-desire is only one vivid, most vivid manifestation. Sex is a changing thing now alive, now quiescent, now fiery, now apparently quite gone. A man says: I don't love my wife any more; I no longer want to sleep with her! But why should he always want to sleep with her? How does he know what other subtle and vital interchange is going on between him and her, making them both whole, in this period when he doesn't want to sleep with her? And she, instead of jibing and saying that all is over and she must find another man and get a divorce—why doesn't she pause, and listen for a new rhythm in her soul, and look for the new movement in the man?

I Join the TAM© Graduate Program

The eight-week TAM group was such a healthy experience for me that I decided to join the TAM Graduate Program. Mel said he had seen me change within eight weeks from a confused, conflicted, sad-faced woman to an upbeat person with hope in her eyes. "You sparkle now," he said with a smile.

I told him TAM had a "graduate" program, which was voluntary for all the participants. The graduate program's objective was different: It was a six-month, once-a-week, group-sharing course from 7:30 P.M. to 9:00 P.M. on Thursdays. It was designed as a refresher course, a weekly reminder to persist in incorporating all the lifestyle changes we had made in our daily lives. That also meant continuing our aerobic exercises. So I joined a separate aerobics rehabilitation program three mornings a week at the same time I joined the TAM Graduate Program. Again, Mel gave me his unconditional support; he also had a memory like an elephant and would remind me of any transgressions, like going off my diet, or "forgetting" a workout session. His concern for my welfare was total, which spurred my recovery.

My original group experience was so positive that I eagerly looked forward to these new once-a-week group sessions. I wasn't disappointed. Everyone in the new group was also moving through the mourning process, each in her or his own way at an individual pace. All of them had advanced from their first "Why me?" depression stage and were struggling toward self-renewal. That was also true of me, for the mourning process is rarely a short eight-week affair. Beginning steps in that process can be achieved in those first weeks, which enabled us to start a new lifestyle and to realize we had the power to make positive things happen. That power had never been lost.

However, now that we had the tools from TAM, to continue in the self-renewal process we had to make use of those tools on a permanent basis. That's why the positive reinforcement of the new six-month graduate group proved so valuable. All of us in that group were struggling to make our new lifestyle permanent. The group had an upbeat spirit from the start, since we had been through the wars and won the battles of the original eight-week program. We all worried about how each member was progressing, and were alert to notice if anyone faltered in following the regimen required for achieving a permanent new lifestyle. If anyone was absent on a Thursday night, we would worry over that fact and ask the person the next time he or she returned what happened and offer helpful suggestions.

There was a pervasive group element of goodwill and a keen awareness of the need a person might have for help (e.g., a suggestion for career improvement, a recommendation for a better health insurance program, a book brought in for a group member concerned about aging, the name of a good marriage counselor, ideas about how to fight against discrimination because of our illness).

Perhaps the greatest compliment the group received came from one of its members, who said, "I had a breast cancer operation before I had my heart attack and my angioplasty. But when a doctor suggested I join a group-sharing program with cancer patients, I decided after attending three sessions I wouldn't continue. It was all so downbeat, everyone was so hopeless. I chose this group instead, because you all have so much spirit and refuse to let anyone get away with feeling hopeless. It's been a privilege to be with you, you've made me feel so much better." She shared these feelings with the group on the last Thursday of the six months.

Shortly after my graduate program ended, I had an extensive physical check-up. When Dr. Sklar finished reading the detailed report, he looked up at me and smiled. "You are a star!" he said with praise in his voice. "You've begun to reverse your heart disease. Your plaque deposits are lower, your cholesterol level and blood pressure are now normal, and so is your weight. You've beaten the odds. You are in many ways healthier than you were at the time you had your heart attack. Continue to function the way you have been doing and you will enjoy a long and quite healthy life."

I was at Stage IV, the self-renewal stage of my mourning process. A new sense of self had emerged, a self that was not in contradiction to my former self, but an extension of that self that has led me in new directions, glistening with exciting new possibilities. I'll be sharing with you the details of that new direction in chapter 10.

9

The Promise in the Future: New Scientific Discoveries That Could Prevent, Heal and Reverse Heart Disease

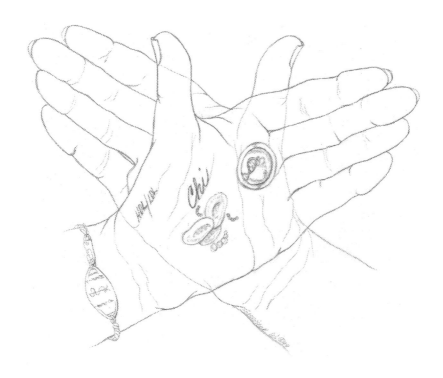

T hree years since my near-death heart attack I feel very fortunate indeed: I have not had a second heart attack. I have kept my weight, cholesterol and blood pressure at normal levels, and no new plaque formations have formed in my arteries. The danger of restenosis seems minimal. (Restenosis is the dangerous reoccurrence in an artery that has been expanded by angioplasty to narrow again, usually in the six to eight months after a heart attack. This further damages the heart.) My heart disease continues to be in a reversal stage. And yet . . .

It would be false to present myself to you as a package of sweetness and light without a worry in the world about how well my heart is functioning. Yes, my heartbeat is normal now, but what about the future? Am I living in a fool's paradise, only to wind up once again as a hospital case? Can I plan for the future? I keep thinking of John Lennon's wry observation, "Life is what happens to you when you are busy making other plans."

It was with these thoughts in mind that I decided to interview Dr. Sklar and Dr. Wexman about the current state of scientific knowledge about heart disease and the latest cutting-edge developments in their field that might reinforce the possibilities of people like myself to lead a long, fulfilling, life while managing our heart disease.

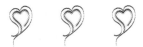

My first interview was with Dr. Sklar:

Q. *Since we're at the cusp of a new millennium, what are the scientific differences in what we know now about heart disease—its prevention, healing and reversal—in contrast to what we knew at the beginning of the century in the year 1900?*

A. • We now know the causes of heart disease.
   • We know we can prevent a lot of heart disease.
   • We know we can treat a lot of heart disease and save millions of lives.

None of these things was true in the early 1900s. People who had heart attacks then just died. People with symptoms of heart disease just lived with those symptoms—there were no treatments, no medicines.

In the early 1900s people died of other things: infections, childbirth, tuberculosis, influenza. The average age when people died was forty-six at the beginning of the century, so women, who are at greatest risk for getting heart disease after menopause, died of other causes before that happened. So heart disease wasn't a big contributor to the death rate in the early 1900s.

But in the year 2000, heart disease is the biggest killer of all adult American men and women. We now live almost twice as long as people did in 1900—seventy-six years is now the average. The effects of aging—combined with lifestyle habits that damage our hearts— kill more men and women today than all other diseases combined. Even so, because of the greater awareness of the population and of physicians and new scientific discoveries, deaths from heart disease have dropped 56 percent since 1950. The lifestyle factors that help prevent such deaths are the drop in cigarette smoking among adults, a greater awareness of healthy diets, and more concern about weight reduction and the need to exercise more, as well as the use of stress reduction techniques.

In the last three decades, particularly, we've made more scientific progress about how to prevent, manage or reverse heart disease than at any other time in history. We've learned to cope with heart attacks through life-saving surgery techniques such as angioplasty and bypass surgery. The medicines today to manage heart disease—such as improved blood-thinning agents, beta blockers, calcium channel blockers and synthetic folic acid—were not available twenty-five years ago. They did not exist when I was in medical school.

There's no single reason that the death rate is going down. The reason is multifactoral. People are becoming more conscious of heart-disease symptoms, so they are coming in to see their doctors earlier and are able to take advantage of the latest medical and surgical techniques before irreversible damage occurs.

Q. *Would you say that in the last five years there have been new, dramatic developments regarding minimizing the damage heart disease creates?*

A. Absolutely. In the last five years there have been two dramatic developments:

1. The most recent development is direct angioplasty, where, if someone comes in having a heart attack, it is now the standard of care in most hospitals that have the ability to do it to take the person directly to the cardiocatheter laboratory, do the angioplasty and that is the end of that heart attack. You have now restored blood flow, and you can do that with a 90 percent or a 95 percent success rate. In this way, you reduce the mortality rate a lot. You get people out of the hospital in several days as opposed to a week, and it is a dramatic difference. If a person comes in with a heart attack, how soon would you give that person angioplasty? Immediately. Makes no difference if it's a man or a woman. That's correct, it makes no difference.

   The ability to do angioplasty on more people with more success and less likelihood of problems down the road is improving. Ten years ago when we did angioplasty there were incidents of near disaster, where you would tear the blood vessel, find a clot in the blood vessel and have to rush to emergency surgery. Something could go wrong and the rate of that happening approached 5 percent. It was a big deal. Today, with new balloons and new catheters, that rate is less than 1 percent. So the rate of acute complication has fallen dramatically.

2. The incidence of recurrence has gone down. If you perform a successful angioplasty, you open a blood vessel. Five years ago, eight years ago, ten years ago, the chance of that specific treatment staying open indefinitely was about 70 percent. On the other hand, 30 percent of the time the blood vessel would close up again. Why wouldn't it stay open? Because the body doesn't like it that you are in there plunging around with a device. It scars badly. Some people scar with big bumpy things, so there is a 30 percent chance of a fibrotic inflammatory process reclosing the blood vessel. This year, with modern-day angioplasty and new clot medicine, that rate of reclosure is less than 15 percent. So the chance of having to come back has been halved.

3. There has been a great advance in bypass surgery techniques in the last few years, just as there has been in angioplasty techniques, and it is saving many more lives. Now successful bypass surgery is being performed without having to use the heart-lung machine!

Many of the complications that relate to bypass surgery relate to stopping the heart and using this bypass machine—the heart-lung machine—to do the function of the heart and lung, and that's hard on the body. It's also hard on the brain and can create blood-clot problems. What's happening in the past several years is that they have learned how to do the same bypass operation, take the veins from the legs or the veins from the chest, and bypass the blockages without stopping the heart, so they're actually operating on a beating heart. Has this been done yet? Absolutely! And that has reduced many of the complications doctors encountered by stopping the heart and using the heart-lung machine. So, I think what's going to happen is that the risk of bypass surgery will continue to fall, as has been happening. And the ability to operate on people who are sicker will improve. Because right now if you have bad lungs or bad vessels, surgery is a big risk. But if you can make the surgery less traumatic, you can reach more people.

In addition, advances in surgery now have drastically modified the size of the incisions in bypass operations. Until recently, incisions were eighteen inches. Now they are a fraction of that size. This is a great boost to a person's self-image, because he or she no longer has a big scar that is a constant reminder of the bypass operation.

Q. *What effect will the new developments in angioplasty and bypass surgery have on longevity?*

A. That's a very tricky area to talk about, because
it all depends on the success rates and on the
selection process. There are groups of people
for whom the only reason to do an operation is
to prevent symptoms, and that includes angioplasty. There are also groups of people for
whom surgery clearly prevents heart attacks,
prevents heart failure by saving muscle, and
therefore saves lives. But you do need to pick
your patients right. And one of the criticisms of
American medicine is that too many people
have operations for insufficient reasons: People
may have operations because the surgeon
wants to do it, or because it will make the
patient feel better, but not to improve longevity
or their mobility. That's a difficult and statisti-
cal discussion that I can't answer simply. I
believe, as with all procedures, that as success
rates improve, applicability widens. And so you
have a better chance of being able to do more
good with less harm, and therefore improve
outlook.

Q. *What are the new culprits contributing to heart
disease?*

A. We're taking a new look at cholesterol. It is
becoming clear that if you have a total cholesterol level of about 200, that can no longer be
considered "good." In fact, we are finding that if
you are looking for reversal of heart disease, or

the prevention of the disease, cholesterols that are very low—170, 160, 150—may make for heart improvement, which a 200 level cannot accomplish.

There is emerging interest in high blood sugars and bacteria that relate to the inflammatory process and how they increase plaque. There's starting to be a lot of scientific evidence that a bacterial infection, specifically one called chlamydia, may be a real heart-disease culprit. If you look at chlamydia—levels of the bacteria in the blood of people with plaque compared to those without plaque, and the resulting antibody levels—people with plaque have higher levels of the bacteria. In Europe, where there is less occurrence of heart disease, we talk about the French paradox. The French eat lots of cheese and drink lots of red wine and it is also true that they have less chlamydia, because they treat their cattle with tetracycline (an antibiotic), whereas here in the United States we treat our cattle with penicillin. Tetracycline kills chlamydia, penicillin does not treat chlamydia. So, maybe that different antibiotic is the way to a man's heart.

The general public believes chlamydia is only a sexual disease that could cause sterility in women. Yes, it is a sexually transmitted disease, but it is much more than that. It's out there, it's everywhere. It's in the food supply, it's a microorganism you can get from just breathing. And people who have chlamydia in their blood vessels are more likely to develop plaque in their blood vessels. It's being very carefully researched, and there is a corollary that makes you think that it might make sense. Until recently everyone thought that ulcers were caused by stress, etc. It turns out that most ulcers are caused by a bacterial infection. It is probably true that stress contributes, but if you have stress but don't have the bacteria, you probably have just a little gastritis and nothing else. But if you have a bacterial infection, it will probably turn to an ulcer, and the way you treat ulcers these days is with antibiotics, so chlamydia, too, could be a hidden culprit.

Q. *Are there any new findings on the differences between men and women regarding heart disease?*

A. The differences are more of a quantitative nature and in degree. That is, the disease looks the same, but women get it later in life because of their hormones, and once they get it they are probably worse off. They have more combined disease conditions. They are more likely to have hypertension, more likely to have smaller blood vessels, more likely to have diabetes. They have smaller blood vessels, so therapies may be more difficult for doctors to perform. It's easier to operate on a big pipe than a small one. Women's symptoms may not be as obvious and may be easily attributed to something else. A woman comes in with lower chest pain and there is a tendency to think that it is lower gastritis and not angina. There may be a delay in diagnosis and therefore a delay in treatment. But it is the same disease men have and it's caused by the same things: smoking, high LDL cholesterol, stress and a sedentary lifestyle.

We use the same techniques to test women for heart disease as we do with men—treadmills, stress tests, those sorts of things—but there is a higher incidence of false positive tests in women. You are not necessarily going to miss heart disease in a woman if you miss a test, but you are more likely to incorrectly diagnose one and to have to go to the next step to prove it's okay. Women's anatomy is different, so if you conduct an echocardiogram or isotope scan, breasts get in the way. They can interfere with the ability to get an acoustic window, and you have to account for that, you have to realize that's an issue.

It is more common for a man to give you the typical story for angina—crushing chest pain down the left arm—and more typical for a woman to experience a burning sensation that's not quite in the center, so you have to be alert that the symptoms are not quite the same. And you have to be aware that if you conduct the same tests, the statistics that apply to those tests differ between men and women.

Q. *Can you single out a specific current research program that may produce the greatest benefit in the future for heart patients?*

A. Yes, the fact that the gene that tells blood vessels to produce more blood vessels is being found. So if you inject the gene that turns on angiogenesis (which is creation of blood vessels), into a mouse or into a person's leg or heart, then you will create new blood vessels. If you can inject the angiogenisis factor into a blood vessel that is blocked, you may not get rid of the blockage, but you may create new channels around it, and that is being researched. There are research programs available right now in the San Francisco Bay Area that allow appropriate candidates to undergo gene therapy. It's being done. What's the prognosis? Good. In some years, it may be as standard to go into the hospital and get injected with the angiogenisis factor as it is to be injected with insulin for diabetes. And it may save your life!

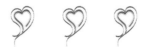

Hope welled in my heart after I interviewed Dr. Sklar. I mean this literally as well as figuratively: He gave me hope that my heart had a great potential for healing and stabilizing itself, so that the damage done to my heart muscle as a consequence of my heart attack would be minimized rather than accelerated in the future—provided, of course, that I maintained my new lifestyle. I felt the desire to plan ahead in my career and personal life for more than just a day at a time (which I had feared doing before because the dark cloud of another heart attack still hovered over me, much as I wanted to deny its existence), a feeling profoundly reinforced by Dr. Sklar's presentation of the present and future scientific findings about heart disease. There had been excitement in Dr. Sklar's voice as he had talked with me. He sounded as if he were in the center of magnificent new scientific developments in heart disease research and practice—new developments that could save millions of lives through new findings in how to prevent, manage and reverse heart disease.

He infected me with his belief that scientists were at the beginning of a new revolution in their ability to eliminate heart disease as today's number-one killer of adult men and women. Instead of being the number-one killer, perhaps it will rank far below cancer by the next decade. This is a bright outlook for people everywhere, and in particular for people who live in heart-disease country. It is an epiphany for the new millennium!

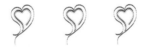

I knew that the codirectors of Cardiology Associates, Drs. Sklar and Wexman, were also coequals in their extensive, up-to-date knowledge of present and cutting-edge developments in cardiology research and practice. So it was with upbeat anticipation that I began my interview with Dr. Wexman shortly after I had interviewed Dr. Sklar. I was not disappointed: his comments and observations were very rich in insight. The questions I asked him centered on issues I had not covered with Dr. Sklar. My summary of the questions and his answers are as follows:

Q. *What new risk factors for heart disease that were unknown or overlooked a decade ago are now considered part of mainstream medicine?*

A. I think of homocysteine first. It is an amino acid in the blood. If you have too much of it, it increases your risk of getting heart disease. If you do not have enough folic acid, B-12 and B-6 vitamins in the diet, then you will have higher levels of homocysteine, and these higher levels will circulate in the bloodstream and damage the very delicate internal cells of the arteries.

It's interesting to note that folic acid was supplemented initially in pregnant women, because high homocysteine levels were known to contribute to birth defects. Doctors then didn't recognize the risk factor of high levels of homocysteine to the heart, and that increasing the use of folic acid and vitamins B-6 and B-12 could significantly lower that risk.

Now a number of good scientific studies show the relationship of high homocysteine to coronary cerebral vascular disease. We are still awaiting a study that shows that by lowering the levels of homocysteine we could change the incidence of death of people with heart disease. That's in the works now.

Q. *In medicine and in science in general, there seems to be a lot of resistance to new ideas. For instance, I read a long article in the* New York Times *a few years ago about how the discoverer* *of the importance of homocysteine levels to heart disease was derided by major scientists who regarded his findings as nonsense (just like Nobel prize winner Linus Pauling was ridiculed for promoting the value of vitamin C). It took at least a couple of decades before these same scientists acknowledged the validity of homocysteine research. Do scientists have a vested interest in resisting new discoveries?*

A. Yes, that happens. On a personal level I received a grant in 1980 to do research in homocysteine. I did the research with my wife and another resident at New York University. What we found was that 16 percent of patients with coronary-artery disease had elevated homocysteine levels, and only 2 percent of the patients with normal coronary arteries had elevated homocysteine levels. That was published in 1984 in the *Journal of the American College of Cardiology*. And I will tell you nobody cared! Because at that time the fashionable body of research was still focusing on cholesterol and lipids (fatty substances). So when I came out west to the University of California, we originally talked about continuing that research out here. But there was little funding and little interest. That's because homocysteine levels were not of interest to pharmaceutical companies since the developments weren't going to result in a new drug that would create big profits. It was going to be treated instead by commonly generic vitamins. Therefore, because there was no product to sell at the end of the research, funding for the re-search was hard to come by.

Now it's all turned around. There has been in the last six years great interest in homo-cysteine. A lot of groups have picked up on it because its now fashionable. There are a large number of articles in cardiology journals on homocysteine.

Or let's take what has been happening in ulcer research. When I went to medical school in the 1970s, scientific wisdom had it that ulcers came from the acid produced in the things you ate. Particular foods were considered the cause of ulcers, and if you eliminated them from your diet, you could avoid ulcers. But scientists have discovered that this is not true. In the last eight or nine years, a small bacteria has been identi-fied as the culprit, not food. So today we are using antibiotics to treat ulcer disease, and they work. But if I had said this when I took my board examination in internal medicine in the 1970s, it would have been the wrong answer. Here again, scientists who had a funding stake in a food-acid connection to ulcer research resisted the now-proven fact that it is a bacteria problem.

Q. *In other words, is it fair to state that "alternative medicine" often becomes mainstream medicine? After all, homocysteine and the new ulcer research were not initially considered forms of traditional medicine. We know that Tai Chi and the Feldenkrais method, acupuncture, vitamins, herbal products—all are considered* *forms of "alternative medicine." Should they be ignored because they are not "traditional medicine" approaches? Should they be considered second-class?*

A. Whether you call a medicine "alternative" or "traditional" or "mainstream" is irrelevant to the fact that if it works, it works—and that's the definition of medicine as we use it. It's the pragmatic value and nothing else that counts. I would hope that we could come to an understanding of the scientific basis of all these different approaches and adopt and incorporate all these good ideas into a common basis of treatment, regardless of the origin of the idea.

Often, the resistance to new ideas is because the status quo tries to maintain the status quo. It's hard to believe, but several years ago there was a controversy about cholesterol. People were trying to decide whether or not cholesterol was a risk factor for coronary heart disease. That controversy has disappeared because the evidence, the scientific data, is now overwhelming and now cholesterol is part of "traditional" medicine. Homocysteine doesn't contradict cholesterol's validity; the researchers are in the same fight together against heart disease.

And when there is talk about herbal medicine being a part of alternative medicine, it's good to remember that 25 percent of the drugs that traditional medicine uses are plant extracts. We do it in a very scientific way: the drugs commonly used in cardiology are from foxglove, which is a derivative of a plant that's been used for medicinal purposes for hundreds of years. Vitamins are now considered part of traditional medicine; only a few years ago they were labeled an alternative medication. Now vitamins are one of the ways we treat homocysteine levels, and vitamin E use seems to lower the incidence of heart disease. Even so, it is a subject still undertaught in medical schools today. We are going to be moving out of the exclusion stage where alternative medicine is considered to be competitive with traditional medicine. Western medicine should be *inclusive,* in the forefront of testing new ideas. Let's study these so-called alternatives well, scientifically, with control groups and without bias. And if they then work, helping to eliminate heart disease is the only criterion that should be used.

Q. *What does the future hold for new developments in understanding the mind/body connections as they relate to heart disease?*

A. I think there is a burgeoning academic interest in a field that we can call psychoneurocardiology. We are now taking a look at things like stress and emotion and heart disease. Research shows that people who have high–hostile-level responses—that is, people who have greater levels of anger and hostility in ways that they deal with the world seem to be in greater risk of heart disease—and heart attacks. An interesting study of hostility in doctors and lawyers demonstrated that lawyers with a low hostility level had a 4 percent or 5 percent twenty-five-year mortality. Doctors with a high hostility rate had a 22 percent to 25 percent twenty-five-year mortality. Low hostility equaled longer life; high hostility shorter life.

The mechanism of the relationship between brain and body is being worked out. We take a look now at people's response to stress and we know that some people create blockages at times of stress ranging from modest to severe. There is a relationship between emotional stress or anger or hostility and blood flow.

We know that heart-disease patients will respond better after surgery if they have a support group. Isolation is clearly a negative response for recovery. The University of Maryland published a study of people in the post-angioplasty stage. They looked at people who were in the low or high hostility range. It turned out that if you were a very hostile person, your restenosis rate—renewed narrowing of an artery, which is very dangerous—was almost twice that of a person with low hostility. So that is an example of a mind/body relationship within the healing process.

I think the graying of American baby boomers will force greater serious thinking about cardiovascular disease. We can expect much more research on the mind/body connection in the future. The baby-boom generation is very receptive to research in this significant field, which has been understudied in the past.

Q. *From what you say, this seems to be a very exciting time for cardiology—a golden age of research and development, which offers great* *hope for heart-disease patients like myself, as well as for people working to prevent heart disease. It seems we are getting a cascade of information on the six o'clock news and in magazines, and newspapers and on the Net about so-called revolutionary "new" cure-alls for heart disease. In your professional opinion, what is the best way for people to separate out the hype from the truth in this information glut about heart disease? What can we believe?*

A.   The pace in which we receive information today has increased tremendously. Reporters of medical events get abstracts and news releases and rarely have time to research the detailed studies about a new drug or a new vitamin or a new surgical technique. It's in their interest to exaggerate the importance of a new finding on heart disease. It's a ratings plus. Just because medical findings about heart problems are reported on the six o'clock news doesn't mean they will turn out to be true. We need to be careful, because there is also the profit incentive, which can give the wrong impression about a drug or a new technique. If a pharmaceutical or surgical company overenthuses about its product, the media may exaggerate its importance, and so the company's stock price then takes a giant jump. So these factors can lead to bad science and bad results.

   I don't know whether you would want to be the first person to try a new technology or drug once you hear about it in the media. You would want to wait and see some long-term results, because sometimes we don't discover side effects of a medicine from the trials reported in a medical study. We see it later from people who are actually using it. That was true about the beta carotenes. It was later discovered they *increased* the risk of former smokers with heart problems, rather than the opposite, which was supposed to happen. So, the beta carotenes today are no longer recommended as an individual supplement.

It's God that packages the carotenes, and not in the way the pharmaceutical companies do. You probably would be better off eating squash, sweet potatoes and green leafy vegetables—these create the result the carotenes were supposed to.

There are no miracle cures for heart disease, so it's best not to rely on just a single study when the media talks about a new discovery, but on the preponderance of studies and from larger populations than are found in one study. In that way, you keep an eye on safety in making decisions.

Q. *What is the best perspective heart-disease patients like myself should use to guide our lives to live as productively as possible?*

A. It's of first importance to focus on the synergy effect for your becoming a stabilized, healthier person. Synergy occurs when you take your cholesterol level seriously and maintain it at a normal level, when you monitor your homocysteines, exercise, eat a low-fat diet, keep a good body weight, lower your stress so that you're not hypertensive, and adhere to your medication.

It's this combination, this interaction of *all* of these components, that will keep you healthy— that's what *synergy* means. There are no fast fixes. This is not a Chinese-menu approach, where you can just pick and choose the item you are interested in and ignore the rest. It all works together, or else it doesn't work at all.

The future of medicine is going to be based on technologies that we can see and things that are across the horizon. I think it's more important to us as individuals to focus more on how many healthy ways we can change our lives by using the *existing* knowledge we have. I would encourage people with heart disease not to wait for promises of some future cure, but to continue to work now with the well-described and well-tested strategies that will reduce their cardiac risk factors in the present. You don't need more science to show you that the synergy approach works. If a person isn't eating a low-fat diet or getting their blood pressure treated or is not exercising, one more study of some new discovery won't make a difference if you are not going to be around to get the value of that study. Whatever you as a person with heart disease face, realize that you are not alone. You are on a road that many others are traveling. There are excellent resources in most communities to help guide you towards a healthier place in your life. You don't have to wait on the future to do that.

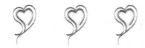

As I reflected on my interviews with Dr. Sklar and Dr. Wexman, after leaving their offices and replaying their tapes, I began to feel a healing in my soul. The fractures in my sense of self that I had been experiencing ever since my heart attack disappeared. The three years I have been living with my heart disease really represented a journey I have been taking—a journey of discovery in which I found new challenges and new opportunities in my life and my career. The perspectives presented to me by Dr. Sklar and Dr. Wexman offered me a takeoff point from which I could explore new horizons, for they diminished much of the fear that had eaten at my soul. They gave me a realistically optimistic view of what the future could hold for my physical well-being, a view valid for millions of others who have experienced heart disease. So now I was ready to fully explore how best I could live my life *with* my heart condition rather than *in spite of* it. As I have said before, I am not my heart disease, but a person who *has* heart disease and must manage it effectively. But I only half-believed that assertion. I sometimes felt I was whistling in the dark by saying it, and all too often my heart disease took priority over who I felt I was. This inhibited my thoughts and actions, particularly about planning for the future.

Now, however, I felt this weight had been lifted from me: I could now be the person I wanted to be at this time in my life, and act accordingly.

So many new possibilities! I'll be sharing them with you in the next, concluding chapter.

10

My Healthy New Sense of Who I Am: The Surprising Gift of My Heart Disease

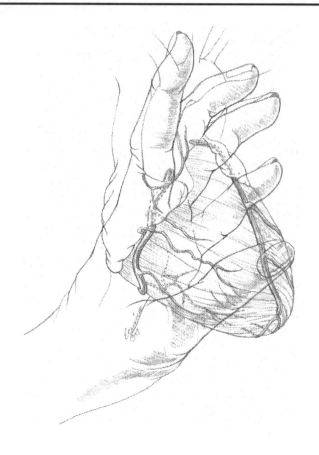

My old self, prior to my heart disease, sits behind a desk. The present me comes into the room and says, "I'd like to introduce myself. I'm the new Pat Krantzler and I wish to acquaint you with who I am today."

The three years since my heart attack seem like a century. Yes, I am a different Pat now, but also the Pat I always had been. Who I am now is still based on the spiritual inheritance I received from my parents. My father was a painter on the Golden Gate Bridge. (When I was a little girl, I thought he owned the bridge because he never had to pay the toll!) My mother was a woman before her time, an accountant before she married, but who by choice wanted to stay home and nurture her family. My mom lost her mother when she was eleven, so she wanted her own family above all else.

To understand who I am now means I must pay attention to my family roots. My mother and father reared me to become a good citizen, to help my neighbors and friends, to be honest, not to cheat, to be helpful in my community. Both my mother and father were kind and understanding and would always reach out to help people more in need than themselves. Their attitude toward the world at large was a consequence of these attitudes. They felt all men and women of all races and places were brothers and sisters. Their hero in politics was Franklin Delano Roosevelt, whose concern for the welfare of everyone was a paramount priority of his administration.

These were the values they imprinted on me, and I'm forever grateful they still live inside of me. It's no accident I became a psychotherapist. Even when I was a child, the first thing that would come into my mind when I woke up each day was not what I was going to do for myself. It was what was it that needed help and my doing it, and what I could do today to help another person.

My parents were religious in a spiritual, ecumenical sense. I can still hear my mother's voice telling me when I was a child that there are many houses of prayer, but there is only one God that shines on all those houses. She told me I was free to visit any church and discover which one felt right for me. It would be my personal choice. She did not believe in a punitive, judgmental God. Her God was kind and understanding. My sister and I prayed each night to a very understanding God, a loving God that would listen to us, our hopes and fears, and would guide us to do the right thing rather than punish us. That spiritual gift from my parents never left me.

As a child I had a great sense of humor and loved to make people laugh. I could break up my family with my impressions. I was considered the family clown, and that was praise, not a put-down. I learned to make people comfortable with my sense of humor.

It's a gentle humor, not a hostile one. My mother used to tell me when I would visit friends, "Be sure to be good company."

That legacy made me friendly and outgoing, and created a thrust inside always to try to make positive things happen, even in the face of adversity. My parents made me feel secure that I was a good person, but also emphasized that I had to make myself personally accountable to continue to be a good person. I could never use a lazy excuse for not doing what I committed myself to do. My parents would catch me every time. That's why I've always been action-oriented; when I say I'll do something, I feel personally responsible to do it. I am accountable to myself.

Before my heart attack, these values were deeply a part of me. Now they are even more important to my sense of self. But now I no longer take them for granted. Instead, I am using them to move in new directions.

People rarely take the opportunity to stop and think about who they are, what they want and how they are going to use the rest of their lives. When we're in our twenties and thirties we think we'll live forever, so there's no reason to think about the future—just living is enough. It's easier to simply drift through life. In our forties and fifties, there's a growing awareness that we are all headed toward an ending. But that's not enough to make us reevaluate who we are and where we are taking our lives. It's just a twinge of awareness. But having a life-threatening disease, such as mine, in one's forties or fifties is really an alarm-bell telling one's soul to wake up and think about what is truly valuable in life, since time may end sooner rather than later.

Ever since my life has become stabilized, thanks to Cardiology Associates and my own efforts, I have learned to use in new ways the values I have lived by. Above all else, I've learned that time is not something I can squander, or drift through, or waste. People talk about "killing time"—a horrifying phrase, for time will kill *us* if we waste it, not vice versa. It will kill us with boredom and mindlessness, two deadly sins. So, to make use of the finite time I now know I have left, I must do what I always wanted to, yet never did, like traveling around the world to foreign lands such as Lucca, Italy, the birthplace of my father, and Ireland, the birthplace of my mother. I've never done so before, because I have always had a great fear of flying. Before my heart attack, I only flew twice in my life—both short trips from San Francisco to Los Angeles. In both cases I was a white-knuckle flyer, and I vowed after my second flight never to fly again.

But in the past nine months I have flown five times, as far as roundtrips to New York and Mexico City. This year I will be flying to Europe for the first time, and I'm eagerly looking forward to it. I have my heart attack to thank for this change in my attitude toward flying. Once you have a heart attack, nothing else will scare you that much. Since I've already faced death, what's to fear from flying? In fact, I'm beginning to enjoy flying now. White knuckles are a thing in my past.

I have been asked by dear friends if I worry each day that I will have another heart attack. My answer is definitely no. Of course, I remember I have had a heart attack when I take my medicine each day and work out at the rehabilitation center three times a week. But that is different from viewing my disease as if it were a killer with a gun waiting just around the corner to murder me. My feeling like a victim, obsessing about another disaster to happen to me, has entirely disappeared from my life. I'm no longer fearful, because I know I am currently paying my dues each day to keep myself healthy. I do my exercises with the greatest regularity. I eat the proper low-fat foods, I make sure my weight is normal, I meditate each day, I get enough sleep. I'm doing everything my doctor wants me to do to keep well. I'm doing more athletic activity than I've ever done before, my muscles are more developed than they were prior to my heart attack; I can lift heavy grocery bags out of my car because my arms are now stronger, and my clothes fit better because my shape is more in tone as I write this. I remember Dr. Sklar saying to me three years ago that I might indeed feel better after my heart attack than the time before I had it. I then thought that he was just trying to give me foolish hope. But now I know it's true. It's true because I no longer take my health for granted. I take personal responsibility to make my good health happen. My goal is to continue to reverse my heart disease, and my regular tests and doctors' evaluations prove this is happening.

My parents gave me a deep sense of security that I would always be able to stand on my own two feet, even if one of them was broken. They made me feel I could carry on, no matter what adversity might hit me. "Don't wallow in what you don't have; take advantage of what you do have," my father used to tell me.

What is now emerging in my life are drives within me that I have never fully acted on before. It's a feeling of becoming what I always was yet never had been. For example, I've been a follower, rather than a leader, most of my life. Yet I had the capacity for leadership: when I was in high school I was elected girl president of some two thousand students. And I also was the featured singer in dance-band concerts. Yet I continued to overlook that drive and was nonassertive and a caregiver, always attending to others' needs instead of my own. But even before my heart attack, the drive to be a leader, not just a follower, occurred with the encouragement of Mel, my present husband. With Mel's reinforcement, I took assertiveness training courses and am now a teacher of assertiveness training. And I went back to college and became a psychotherapist (which I once thought was an impossible dream).

So the grounding was there in my personality to become more of a leader than a follower. But it's taken my heart disease to make me move in the new direction of wanting to fulfill my drive to be a leader. It's given me a new sense of purpose in my life. I feel a powerful need to be in the forefront of getting my message across, not only to people next door, or neighbors, or in my personal counseling practice, but all over the world. It means establishing new career directions in my life.

The Message of My New Career as a Psychocardiologist

What message do I want to send to the world? It's my newly emerged passionate commitment to help people recover from heart disease, to reverse it and lead full, productive lives, even though the disease needs to be monitored for the rest of one's life. Indeed, one of my first steps in actualizing this new calling in my life is by writing this book, essential to healing heart disease. It offers a psychological approach to severe medical problems. It demonstrates that one can prevail over heart disease, rather than be permanently traumatized by it. I call my approach to heart disease a "psycho-cardiology" approach. This approach acknowledges the need for the best medical care one can get, but at the same time emphasizes the equal need for psychological care, if one is to help men and women overcome the mental and physical effects of a damaged heart.

It may seem strange to read of my new commitment to work with heart-disease patients since I mentioned in the first chapter my fear of hospitals and physical disease (as opposed to psychological concerns) and doctors and medicine (before my heart attack, medicine and pills were anathema to me). But there is no contradiction. Rather, it's a new development in my life. I can use in new ways skills that I've practiced with clients for the past fifteen years, transferable skill I now can use counseling groups of heart-disease patients. I have lost my fear of doctors, hospitals, physical illness and medicine. My own heart disease has been my greatest teacher. It's taught me to come to terms with my own physical illness, and I now regard doctors, hospitals and medicine as components that save lives. Before I suffered a heart attack, I still held my childhood view of my mother's physical illness as something that inevitably led to death. That created my fear of any physical illness and my tendency to take on clients who only

needed help solving interpersonal-relationship problems of a nonphysical disease nature.

That attitude of mine has completely vanished
today. But I feel it's made me uniquely qualified to be
empathic and sensitive to the fears and emotional
fragility of people with a life-threatening disease
such as mine. And because of the traumatic, emotionally shattering effect such a life-threatening disease has on a person's psyche, the most skillful kind
of psychological counseling could be of greatest help
in renewing one's life instead of becoming overwhelmed by depression. Since I've been-there-done-
that, and am also a psychological counselor who has
always enjoyed working with groups, I feel I can
make a real contribution to the emotional welfare of
heart-disease patients whose severe psychological
problems have not been addressed. It's the quality of
one's life that needs saving, along with the physical
life of a heart patient. It matters little if the body is
patched up but the soul remains mired in depression
for the rest of one's life.

I would like to focus my counseling work primarily
on women heart patients. This does not mean that
mixed groups of men and women are not useful, too.
But I believe women have special psychological problems that need to be exclusively focused on that men
do not have (men have other problems of importance
that need to be considered, but in groups of their
own or in mixed groups).

My new, passionate desire to help such women
attain self-renewal is another "seed beneath the
snow" that always has lived inside of me, but is now
emerging in this form. I have always felt, since I was
a young girl, that it was very unfair of society to treat

women as second-class citizens. Even when I was in high school, I was the person who would reach out to new women students looking vulnerable in coming to school for the first time, welcome them, make them feel more comfortable, ask them to have lunch with me—it was because I cared. I always wanted to help women who seemed to need help. So it's really no accident that this thrust to help women is now emerging in this form. For who could feel more vulnerable than a woman with heart disease?

I now view myself as a psychological educator and therapist in the new field of psychocardiology (the heart and mind connection). Millions of women have experienced heart disease and have received the medical attention they need to save their physical lives. What they need, but do not receive, is the focused psychological attention that will help them understand their emotions arising from their heart disease. Some women remain depressed, even suicidal, because they believe they have lost forever their ability to make positive things happen in their lives. They wear the costume of a victim and never take it off.

I have a great belief in the ability women (all women) have to overcome adversity and experience new transformations. All they need is to be provided with the insight, information and skills to triumph over a profound trauma.

The All-Women's Psychocardiology Counseling Group

My first step in my new career took place six months ago. At that time I established a group of twelve women, all who recently had either a bypass operation or angioplasty. I also included women who were on the cusp of a heart attack and were on a regimen of medicine, diet and exercise to prevent an attack from happening. They met for twelve sessions, on Wednesday evenings from 7:30 P.M. to 9:00 P.M. I was the group leader. I told them I was not a guru, but a catalyst who wanted them to share their deepest concerns about their illness, to voice unspoken thoughts that they had hidden even from their loved ones. They would discover they are not alone in their feelings and struggles: They would hear others in the group voice similar concerns. All members of the group had a common goal, to cope with their terrible feelings of loss: the loss of their old healthy selves, who took their life for granted rather than worrying about what the next hour, let alone the next day, would bring.

At my first session, I congratulated them on joining the group. It was an act of courage on their part to make the effort to face up to their sense of loss by joining the group. They would discover that the group members would reinforce their courage to overcome their difficulties. All of the members of the group were in the same boat and they consequently had great empathy, compassion and concern for each member's welfare. In that sense, I was no different from any group member. I, too, was one of them. I was "different" only in the sense that I had the group-counseling skills to elicit the strengths inherent in each person and help them cope with their weak-nesses. And since I was also a woman, the group felt the counseling sessions were a safe place to share the widest range of what they were feeling. There were no men present, so the women felt less inhibited.

My psychocardiology approach focused on a central theme. It was "The Healing Process of Mourning." As I explained in chapter 8, mourning takes place after experiencing a profound personal loss, like the death of a loved one or the death of a relationship (divorce). It also occurs after the loss of the "old self" a person experiences after a heart attack. Mourning is a healthy process that takes place over time. In the beginning, it involves feeling very depressed, and the movement from depression to self-renewal occurs when the mourning process runs its course.

When I explained this fact to the members of my group at the first session, the sad aura that covered their faces when they first sat down in the room began to lift as they were given scientific hope that they could once again feel like persons of worth and competency. The mourning process could give them a future.

After they identified themselves, I asked them what they have been feeling repeatedly after they experienced heart disease. Here are their answers:

- "I feel overwhelmed."
- "Everything is so hopeless."
- "I feel helpless."
- "I'm afraid about what might happen next."
- "I'm weepy most of the time."
- "Nothing matters, I have no interest in anything."
- "I have lost all my energy."
- "I can't sleep nights."
- "I'm so irritable."
- "I'm angry at the world."
- "I'm so anxious about everything."

- "I feel so lost."
- "I can't concentrate anymore."

All of the members of the group were feeling a combination of those feelings most of the time since they had heart disease—feelings that never seemed to go away for weeks on end, feelings that were present at this first session.

When I informed them these were the symptoms of clinical depression, they were surprised. They thought they had "the blues," a temporary upset, and nothing more. Depression—if not dealt with or unknown to the person experiencing it—can be one of the most deadly illnesses. It particularly affects women. An estimated 25 percent of all women will undergo clinical depression at some time in their lives. Depression has been linked to heart disease as being even a riskier factor than smoking or cholesterol. Depressed people are twice as likely as the nondepressed average person to have a heart attack. People who are depressed have a 20 percent greater increase in plaque than nondepressed persons. Depression is a killer.

That's the dark side of depression. The bright side of depression (if depression is an inevitable initial consequence of heart disease rather than genetically based) is that it can be part of the beginning stage of the mourning process outlined in chapter 8. Since this was the case with this group, they now could see that their future was not hopeless. I found in my group that depression sometimes occurs when a person has a lot of held—in anger over their situation. Once I helped them get in touch with their anger, they began to heal.

Most women with heart disease are afflicted with one unique quality that men do not have. That is the feeling of guilt, GUILT in capital letters. It is the guilt of no longer being able to be the caregiver they were before the heart attack. Even though many important, valuable changes have taken place in our culture since the women's revolution began in the late 1960s, the belief that a woman is the family caregiver, not the man, remains constant. While men have indeed contributed more in the way of helping with household duties, whether a partner is sick or not, that function is still minimal. The woman is the glue that holds a family together. That is an unspoken acknowledgement in family life. When that glue dries up, family life can unravel.

This feeling of losing this major part of one's sense of self was shared by all the members of the group, who felt they were no longer whole persons now that they could no longer be the caregiver to their family that they were before their heart disease occurred. Consequently they now were carrying a heavy burden of personal guilt on their shoulders, because they could no longer measure up to the expectations of their family—expectations of caregiving that could no longer be taken for granted.

This was a central issue that the members of the group raised and dealt with throughout our twelve sessions. Here are some of the ways the group members expressed their guilt feelings:

- "I feel I've disappointed my family."
- "It's my fault I can't help the family. I should have stopped smoking long ago."
- "I hate to ask my husband to go grocery shopping.

I always did the shopping before. I feel I haven't the right to ask him."
- "I used to spend the afternoons playing with my grandchildren at the park. They look so disappointed when I tell them I can't do that now. I cry when they leave my room."
- "When I tell my son to do the laundry he looks at me as if I were punishing him."
- "I find it hard to buy good Christmas gifts now, because I always worked part-time before, but I can't now. It makes me feel so bad."
- "I feel my husband is always looking at my surgical scar."
- "I can't plan meals for my family anymore. I'm a good cook and the family always enjoyed my baking. Now my daughter has to cook and I know she resents it, even if she doesn't say anything about it."
- "I earned as much as my husband, but I can't work now. I know he's angry with me, he's so silent."

Over twelve weeks, the members of the group began to see themselves in a new light. They realized they weren't born to be service industries, that they had a right to expect mutuality from their families. A committed relationship means asking for help when it's needed as well as giving it. Being a care-receiver is equally valid as being a caregiver. Being able to *accept* caregiving is as much a skill as caregiving is.

My working with this group was one of the best experiences in my life. All of them felt themselves working through their individual mourning process successfully as a consequence of the twelve sessions.

The success of this group proved to me that the calling I had followed to work with women heart-disease patients was the right choice.

I was so proud of the strength these women exhibited. They did not hide their deepest feelings about themselves, their spouse or partner, their children, or relatives—feelings both negative and positive. Women usually are more comfortable expressing their emotions than men are; they don't feel inferior if they say they are sad or scared or vulnerable or feel like crying. Men feel as deeply as women about their heart problems, but often find it very difficult to express themselves in a group. They feel as if their manhood is attacked if they acknowledge their vulnerability. Women have a stronger sense of self in that regard. They are more comfortable in their femininity than men are in their masculinity.

Women's Heart Disease Is Political as Well as Personal

My own heart disease has alerted me to the relative neglect of women in heart-disease research studies and in educating the public about heart disease as the number-one killer of women. Prevention of heart disease in women should be a top priority of our government.

I always keep in mind that the government is not something separate from us. My parents taught me that we, the general public, are the government and therefore have a right to demand positive action from it. That's why I was happy to see recently a full-page ad sponsored by the American Heart Association in the *New York Times.* The ad pointed out that federal funding of heart-disease research projects has decreased rather than increased in recent years, in spite of the need for more funding, since heart disease is the number-one killer in our country. I have written to our congresspersons urging them to support greater funding, and sent them the tear sheet of that American Heart Association ad, which said, "If you knew how underfunded heart disease and stroke research was, you'd have chest pains."

I have seen how a political-action approach to breast cancer can create a successful health campaign. Breast-cancer research funding has increased significantly since millions of women have begun campaigning to make that happen. If that can happen with breast cancer, it can happen with heart disease. The contrast is striking: breast cancer kills 46,000 women each year, but heart disease kills 250,000! When women speak out, we can be heard.

In the past there has been a neglect of women in heart-disease research and in identifying the diagnostic differences between men's and women's symptoms of a potential heart problem. This situation is now changing because of the aging of the baby-boomer generation and many more women experiencing menopause. Before menopause, fewer women have heart attacks because they are protected with estrogen. But recent data reveals that estrogen protection decreases significantly after menopause, so women today are at greater risk than men for having heart attacks from age of thirty-eight and older. The focus in the past was always on men, because they experienced far more heart attacks than women when they were in their thirties or forties. Now the situation is changing, with women in their post-menopausal years suffering heart attacks more frequently than men. (Our society now has 50 million women age fifty and older, the time of greatest risk for women's heart disease.) We women today are becoming more assertive because of that fact. We're saying, "Attention must be paid!"

The Internet, which is an invaluable source of help to people with heart disease, enabling us to bond through chat rooms, unfortunately can also work against us. That's because access through the Internet to the medical backgrounds of all persons is available for a modest price to anyone wishing to gain the information. The *New York Times* recently reported this alarming fact. Employers are still reluctant to hire people with a heart-problem background, even though they may be healthy now and could easily perform most jobs successfully. Employers who wish to discriminate against heart-disease patients can use such information either to refuse to hire us or to fire people with a heart-disease background. One of the ways we women with a heart-disease background can remedy this appalling situation is to engage in organizations that fight such discrimination.

I have not yet discussed the problem that endangers our lives the most—the enormous cost of medical care. An angioplasty costs fifteen thousand to twenty thousand dollars and bypass surgery twice as much. Subsequent care adds another mountain of cost. For people younger than sixty-five who do not have Medicare, the cost of heart-disease medical care can and does shatter many families' traditional way of life. It bankrupts them. And 45 million men and women have no health insurance whatsoever. How many unnecessary heart-attack deaths have occurred among this part of the population unable to pay for life-saving health care?

HMOs, in their present form, unfortunately have not been the answer to this truly desperate situation. In fact, there is a national outcry from doctors and patients who subscribe to HMOs against HMO practices. A recent study by the reputable Henry J. Kaiser Family Foundation reports that nine out of ten doctors said they have patients who have been denied care by an HMO.

The health of our population, all 270 million of us, is a precious national resource. Improving our health care arrangements is a political issue, and since each of us *is* the government, we can, if we have the dedication, vastly improve the current situation.

I've never been politically active before in the sense of joining a political party or fighting for a specific national cause. I thought I did my duty as a good citizen by voting. I always attended parent-teachers association meetings when my children were young, and participated in local neighborhood watch organizations. But that was the extent of my "political" concerns before my heart attack. My view of politics now has expanded as a result of my new psychocardiology career.

But am I really so different in becoming actively concerned about national health issues? The more I think about this new dimension on my life, the more I see it as a social inheritance from my parents. The values they imprinted on me were those of wanting society to provide a decent life for everyone. So isn't my desire for better health care and my active engagement in organizations to make that possible an elaboration on their beliefs? In acting as I do today, I am motivated by my parents' value system.

The Spiritual Gift of My Heart Disease

I've always been a religious person, not only in a churchgoing way, but also in a spiritual way. As I mentioned earlier in this chapter, that legacy was handed down to me from my parents. They believed in a kind, loving, understanding God, and that belief has lived in my soul ever since childhood. It is that God who I believe has given me the call to help as many people as possible renew their lives, to regard their heart disease as an opportunity for self-renewal as kinder, more compassionate human beings. That's the spiritual gift my heart disease has given me, and it is a gift accessible to every woman and man with a heart problem, if only they will reach for it—the gift of connectinhg with the world in a more empathetic way.

On this spiritual foundation I conclude my book. Living through my heart attack and reversing my heart disease, I believe, are gifts from God just as much as medicine. It is in that conjoining of God and medicine that I wish to share with you the spiritual gift—the six profound learning experiences my heart disease gave me:

- I am grateful and thankful that I lived and didn't die from my heart attack. My religious belief and medical technology made that happen.
- I welcome and enjoy the gift of each new day. I no longer take a new day for granted.

- I realize that life is an affair of people, not of things. It is to be lived, not feared.
- I feel closer to my children and my sister than ever before.
- Kindness, empathy, courage and hope are the sources of our personal power. These fundamentals are the ground to stand on, for money and fame are quicksand when we have been visited by death.
- My parents are always with me, for their spirit has never died. That spirit moves me to want to make this precious world of ours a better place in which to live.

Index

guilt (personal), lifting,
195–96
"Healing Process of
Mourning," 193
political aspect of heart
disease, 197–201
psychocardiologist, new
career as, 188–97
spiritual gift, 201–2
values, using in new ways,
183–88
women's psychocardiology
counseling group,
191–97
Graduate Program, Total
Atherosclerosis
Management (TAM), 66,
153–56
group-support and sharing,
66, 71, 87–89, 111, 114.
See also emotional
support; mourning
process
guilt (personal), lifting, 195–96
"guilty pleasures," 125

H
HDL (good) cholesterol, 98–99,
102–3
"Healing Process of Mourning,"
193
heart attack experience, 3–11.
See also heart disease
facts; home from the
hospital; hospitalization
heart disease facts, 43–57
age and risks, 55, 96, 102
American Heart Association
Web site, 52–53
aspirin, 45
atheromatous plaque
(figure), 41
atherosclerosis, 46, 47, 48,
52
blood pressure, 20, 46,
72, 98, 105
blood thinners, 45

breast cancer versus, 54,
101
cholesterol rates, 46, 98–99,
102–3, 105, 165–67
coronary heart disease,
43–44
curing versus managing,
43–48
deaths from, 52, 56, 161–62
diagnosing, 55–56
genetic factors, 45, 96, 102
lifestyle changes, need for,
30, 31–32, 44–48
managing versus curing,
43–48
for men, 52, 53, 54, 55
menopause and, 52, 55,
99–100
*Mosby's Medical, Nursing
and Allied Health
Dictionary,* 51–52
plaque (fatty-deposit),
29–30, 41
reversing, 43–45
smoking, 20, 30, 44, 55,
97–98, 102, 104–5,
109–12
studies of, 54, 159–80
symptoms, 3–5, 54, 55–56,
57
Total Atherosclerosis
Management (TAM)
Program, 46–51, 61–91
for women, 52, 53–57,
167–68
See also gifts of heart
disease; heart attack
experience; lifestyle
changes; medications;
mourning process; risk
factors; scientific
discoveries; Total
Atherosclerosis
Management (TAM)
Program
Henry J. Kaiser Family
Foundation, 200

S

Sadler, Alan, on stress management (TAM Program), 61, 77–81, 117
sadness, 130–31
scientific discoveries, 159–80
  alternative medicine, 173–75
  angiogenesis factor, 168–69
  angioplasty, 17, 29–30, 161, 162–63, 165
  bypass surgery, 161, 163–64, 165
  chlamydia, 166–67
  cholesterol, 165–67
  deaths from heart disease, 52, 56, 161–62
  folic acid, 171
  French paradox, 166
  homocysteine, 171–73
  longevity, 165
  medications, 161
  mind/body connections, 175–76
  1900s, discoveries since, 160–62
  risk factors, 171
  surgery, 161, 162–64
  synergy effect for health, 178–79
  truth versus hype, 177–78
  women versus men, 167–68
secondary smoke as risk factor, 98, 112
sedentary lifestyle as risk factor, 99, 103
self-fulfilling prophecies, 72
self-image, building. See Feldenkrais Method; Tai Chi
"Self-Renewal" stage, 140, 141–46, 156
sexual relations, 146–53
shock, 137, 138–39
Shulman, Alix Kates, on devotion, 150

"silent killer" (hypertension), 20, 46, 72, 98, 105
Sklar, Joel
  on angiogenesis factor, 168–69
  on angioplasty, 29–30
  on chlamydia, 166–67
  on cholesterol, 165–67
  as Codirector of Cardiology Associates, 61, 64–67
  on longevity, 165
  on managing versus curing disease, 43–46, 57
  on minimizing damage from heart disease, 162–64
  on scientific discoveries, 160–62
  on sex and heart disease, 147–48
  on smoking, 97–98, 109, 110
  on women versus men, 167–68
smoking
  giving up, 109–12
  as risk factor, 20, 30, 44, 55, 97–98, 102, 104–5
spiritual gift of heart disease, 201–2
spouse's support for recovery, 32–33, 39, 154
Stilwell, Joseph Warren, on adversity, 35
stress
  acute versus chronic, 70
  management, 66, 76–81, 117
  as risk factor, 100, 106
stuck in stages, being, 144–45
studies of heart disease, 54. See also scientific discoveries
substitution versus deprivation, 92, 111–12
Successful Aging (Rowe and Kahn), 96

W

walking after hospitalization, 27

Web site, American Heart Association, 52–53

weight as risk factor, 99, 103

Wexman, Mark
  on alternative medicine, 173–75
  as Codirector of Cardiology Associates, 61, 64, 89–92
  on folic acid, 171
  on homocysteine, 171–73
  on mind/body connections, 175–76
  on synergy effect for health, 178–79
  on truth versus hype, 177–78

"Why Me?" stage, 137, 138–39

women and heart disease, 52, 53–57, 167–68

women's psychocardiology counseling group, 191–97

"wounded healer," 39–40. *See also* home from the hospital

A Note to the Reader

The next step after reading a book whose ideas seem helpful is to put those ideas into practice. To help you in that endeavor, feel free to contact me:

Pat Biondi Krantzler
Psychocardiologist Counselor
P.O. Box 6213
San Rafael, CA 94903
fax: (415) 454-1672
email: *MELKR@aol.com*

More from the *Chicken Soup for the Soul*® Series

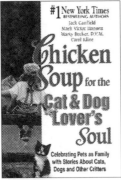
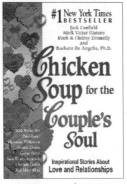
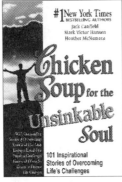
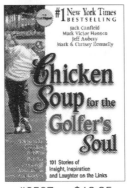
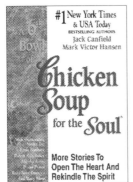